an introduction to:

TAI CHI

and Taoist Energy Meditation.

by

Gary Khor

A BOOBOOK

BOOBOOK PUBLICATIONS

AUSTRALIAN ACADEMY OF TAI CHI

NEW SOUTH WALES (HEAD OFFICE)	PO Box 1327, Crows Nest, NSW 2065 Tel. (02) 929 7433
QUEENSLAND	PO Box 597, Fortitude Valley, QLD 4006 Tel. (07) 358 1955
VICTORIA	PO Box 343, Richmond, VIC 3121 Tel. (03) 428 0600
WESTERN AUSTRALIA	PO Box 1065, Booragoon, WA 6154 Tel. (09) 330 1849
SOUTH AUSTRALIA	GPO Box 1306, Adelaide, SA 5001 Tel. (08) 272 0499
CANBERRA	Tel. (062) 82 5171
NEWCASTLE	Tel. (049) 49 7927
WOLLONGONG	Tel. (042) 67 3454

Call the number in your area for information on class locations, class times, wall charts, music cassettes, video cassetes and instruction tapes.

First published in 1981 by Boobook Publications,
P.O. box 238, Balgowlah, N.S.W. 2093, Australia.

U.S. Distribution: China Books and Periodicals
2929 24th Street, San Francisco, CA 94110

Printed and typeset in Australia by
Southwood Press, Marrickville.

National Library of Australia
Cataloguing-in-Publication entry

Khor, Gary, 1947 —
Tai chi and Taoist energy meditation.

ISBN 0 908121 05 9.

1. T'ai chi ch'uän. I. Title.

796.8'155

Introduction

The purpose of this beginner's manual is to introduce you to the art of Tai Chi and Taoist energy meditation in the most simple and concise way.

It does not matter how old you are or how out of condition you may be; this non-strenuous and non-exertive art is suitable for all. With a little patience and enthusiasm you can master and enjoy its flowing movements and relaxing effects.

As a daily health maintenance system Tai Chi has proved invaluable to the Chinese for generations, and for city dwellers is one of the most effective stress and tension relievers. However, it is also indispensable as a supplementary body tuning system for other sports and hobbies.

Although this book contains all the information necessary for a basic introduction to Tai Chi and Taoist energy meditation, you are advised to seek out an experienced teacher for further instruction.

For centuries the Chinese jealously guarded their health secrets. It is only recently that such knowledge has become more accessible, and it is my hope that this book will add to the growing interest in Chinese healing arts.

What is Tai Chi?

Tai Chi is a form of moving meditation which has been practised in China for thousands of years. Based on a continuous flowing movement the exercise is performed in slow motion and co-ordinated with deep diaphragmatic breathing.

Visually it resembles an effortless dance, but in reality every movement is precise and is performed with a great deal of internal strength.

Through the practice of the art one seeks to harmonise internal energy by promoting a balance between body and mind.

The art and philosophy of Tai Chi is derived from three main sources — the collective philosophies of the Chinese, Shaolin martial art and the study of nature. It is unique among the world's exercise systems in that it is also a living philosophy, dynamic meditation, natural healing system and a self defence art.

Although Tai Chi's benefits are numerous, it is best known for its relaxing and calming effects. Its swimming and weaving motions soothe tired and overstimulated nerves and loosen tense muscles. Modern living conditions subject us to immense stress, leaving us drained at the end of each day. Tai Chi's flowing movements and energy meditation have the therapeutic effect of slowing down the mind and refreshing the body.

As a healing art, it is widely used by the Chinese to treat conditions of stress, depression, mental strain, listlessness, chronic indigestion, insomnia, arthritis, rheumatism, obesity and so on. Because of its preventive and therapeutic properties, it is common practice for Chinese doctors to prescribe Tai Chi as part of the treatment for ailing and convalescing patients. In fact many Chinese doctors are Tai Chi practitioners themselves.

Although the art is suitable for all ages, it is particularly popular with the older Chinese because of its non-exertive and non-strenuous movements — it is practised for recreation, relaxation, body fitness and mental alertness. It is not uncommon for visitors to the East to be captivated by the sight of groups of Tai Chi practitioners going through their rhythmic movements each morning at sunrise in parks and on rooftops.

Tai Chi is also taught to children at school to relax and refresh them after periods of school lessons.

On the artistic level, Tai Chi movements have been used creatively to enhance the flow and movement of dancers, actors, musicians and masseurs.

Why exercise?

Traditionally the basic quest for survival provided the human body with enough exercise. The caveman's nomadic existence and regular hunting forays kept his body active and fit; agricultural societies provided enough exercise through daily routines. With the advent of the Industrial Revolution, the natural body maintenance system was eliminated.

The body thrives on exercise and without it will deteriorate — just like a car, the body needs proper maintenance and constant usage to keep it running smoothly. Regular exercise keeps the body fit and the mind alive, increasing the capacity for activity and the ability to enjoy life and leisure.

However, there is one big obstacle. Exercises tend to become dull and boring, especially when they require no active mental participation. How often have you rushed out to join a new exercise class with great enthusiasm, only to drop out once the novelty has worn off? The generally accepted concept of exercise in the Western world is hard and vigorous physical exertion. Unfortunately this often results in painful injury, permanent damage or uneven bodily development.

Tai Chi is a masterpiece of body and mind co-ordination. The mind visualises each and every movement while the body gives physical expression to that mental image. For example, in the movement called **"Grasping the Bird's Tail"**, the mind visualises the open left palm supporting a delicate little bird, while the right palm strokes its head, runs down its back and through to its tail. As the bird flies away the body rotates to follow its flight.

The active participation of the mind with the body movements creates a sense of softness and sensitivity resulting in a very pleasant flowing meditation.

Tai Chi movements are designed to tone, stretch and exercise every muscle in the body and use the principles of non-exertion and internal energy circulation. The body is put through intricate twisting, gyrating and stretching motions in all directions, based on the natural mobility of the joints and muscles. Many of these movements evolved from the study of animals and nature, and were refined over hundreds of years into precise sets of exercises.

Moving meditation

In its normal state the mind is a constant source of mental activity, a never-ending network of thought associations. Just stop for a moment and try to think of nothing.

Impossible, isn't it?

In the endless sea of thoughts the mind gets no rest. Even in sleep, unfinished business during the day is played out in dream fantasies. In stressful situations such as broken relationships, or financial predicaments, the turmoil is increased. Fortunately we have natural safety valves such as sleep, leisure, sports, hobbies and to a certain extent, daily chores. However, residue pressure continues to build up inside. Meditation has proved to be one of the most effective ways of relieving this pressure.

In essence, meditation consists of concentration and relaxation; the mind focusing on an object while the body relaxes in a comfortable position. This is further enhanced by a passive attitude and a quiet environment.

The basic aim is to silence the thinking mind (the inner chatter) and shift the awareness from the rational to the intuitive mode of consciousness.

In many forms of meditation this silencing of the rational mind is achieved by concentrating one's attention on a single item, like one's breathing, the sound of a mantra, or the visual image of a mandala.

Tai Chi is one of the more pleasurable forms of meditation. Its flowing movements and mental visualization give it an extra dimension which is not present in the static forms of meditation.

As movement is the natural state of living things, it is therefore much easier to meditate this way than to strike up a static pose. Because of its flowing nature, Tai Chi is called ''Moving Meditation'' or ''Meditation in Motion''.

In the practice of Tai Chi there is a central theme that runs through the whole system — the cultivation, storage and circulation of the ''Chi'' or intrinsic energy. In Chinese, the circulation of Chi is called ''Chi Kung'' or energy meditation.

Chi

The single most important and profound concept in the Chinese health system is the circulation of Chi. Simply translated it means energy or life-breath, but it has been variously defined as vital force, intrinsic energy or bio-electricity.

It is an intangible power directly linked to deep rhythmical breathing. Philosophically, Chi is the equivalent of the spiritualist's ether or the scientist's matter-energy theory. The Chinese believe that Chi fills the universe and it neither increases nor diminishes.

Chi is stored in the tan tien, or psychic centre; an area about seven centimetres below the navel. It is circulated throughout the body by the meridian system. According to acupuncture theory the meridian system carries Chi and blood to the organs.

Our personal Chi is inseparable from the Chi of the universe and continually interchanges with it — that is the essence of life, a reciprocal flowing back and forth. When the flow is strong and unhindered, we are healthy; a slight reduction causes sickness; if the flow stops temporarily we become unconscious; if the flow stops completely and irreversibly, we die.

In Tai Chi practise the Chi is lowered to the tan tien, thus lowering one's centre of gravity and establishing a more stable position. At this point, the mind and body become peaceful and tranquil, and all movements become graceful and harmonious.

The living philosophy

Tai Chi derives its philosophical principles from the I Ching or Book of Changes, one of the oldest Chinese books of wisdom, and also from the natural sciences of the Taoist.

The Yin Yang theory

A basic Taoist concept is that the universe is created through the interaction of two forces, the Yin and Yang. Diagrammatically this is represented by a circle divided into two equal parts by a serpentine line. These two halves represent the two polarities in everything. For example, in sex there is male and female, in temperature hot and cold, in time day and night and so on. This principle is embodied in the Tai Chi movements. Each movement is a succession of an opposite action, so that the hand which is above descends and the hand which is below, rises. No movement is complete in itself; it is always moving towards its opposite. The end of one movement is the beginning of another.

The organic universe

The Taoist views the universe as an organic whole; everything in it is related. Man is but one small piece of the whole and in order to grow to his full potential he must observe the laws of nature.

The true art of living is to be able to flow with the Tao, that is the way of nature. For example, everything in the universe is constantly changing and renewing itself in a cyclical pattern. This process is easily observed in the changing seasons. The freshness of Spring gradually changes into the long hot Summer. Summer fades into the colourful Autumn. Autumn loses its leaves and gives way to the cold Winter, and Winter slowly but surely melts into the glorious Spring, completing the cycle.

Just like the changing seasons, Tai Chi movements are forever changing. No posture is held — it is a continuous flow, each posture melting away as soon as it is formed.

This follows the Taoist philosophy that life is not permanent, it is forever changing. Life is not static, for whatever is static is dead.

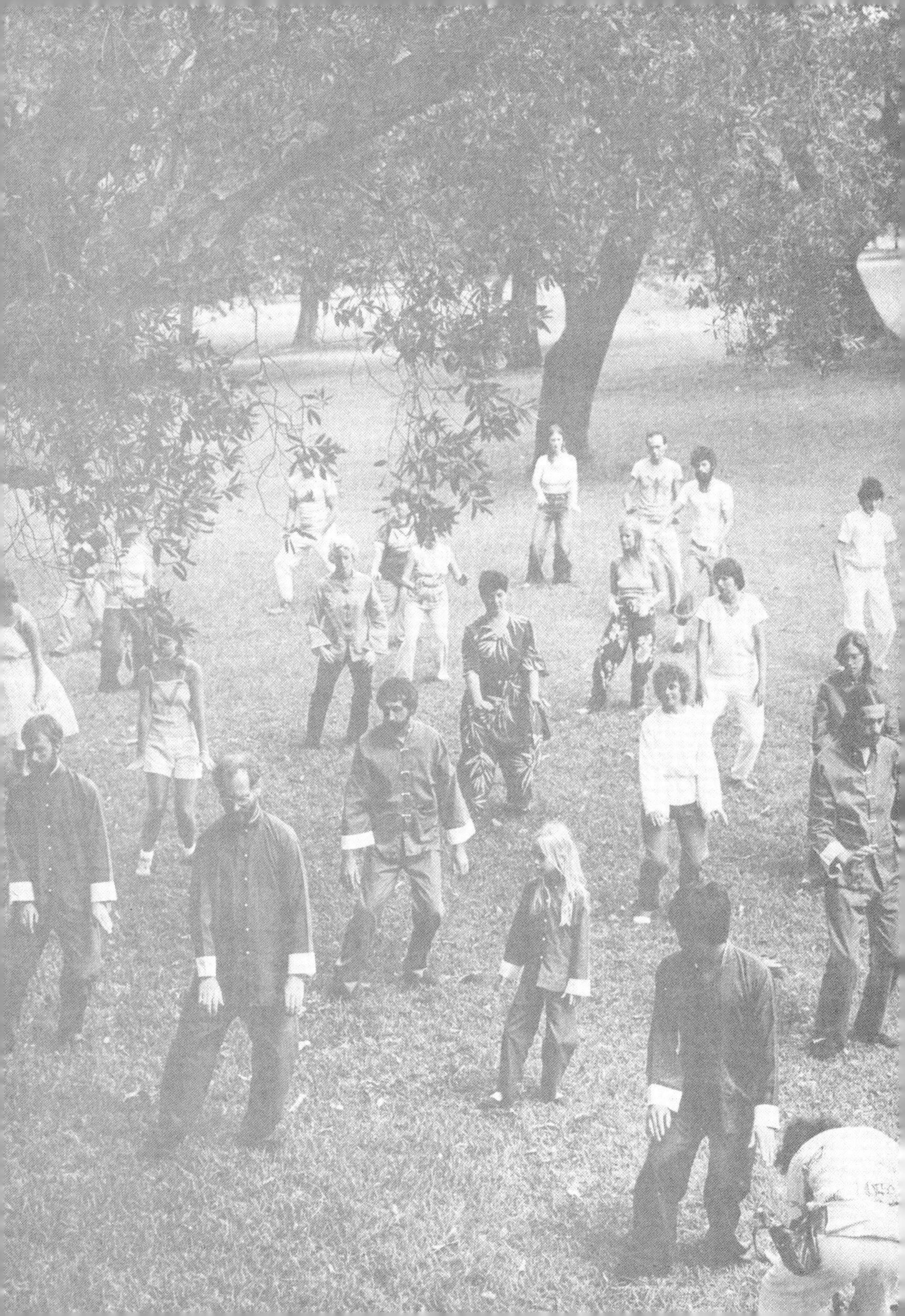

Table of movements

Essential principles in practising Tai Chi

The following key points must be closely observed:

1. Relaxation	Be soft and yielding. Exert no strength.
2. Concentration	Let the mind direct each movement.
3. Meditation	Move slowly with even tempo, describing circles in continuous flow.
4. Harmony	Move all parts of the body as one, with balance and co-ordination.
5. Breathing	Breathe naturally through the nose into the abdomen (tan tien). With the abdomen relaxed, tranquility will prevail.

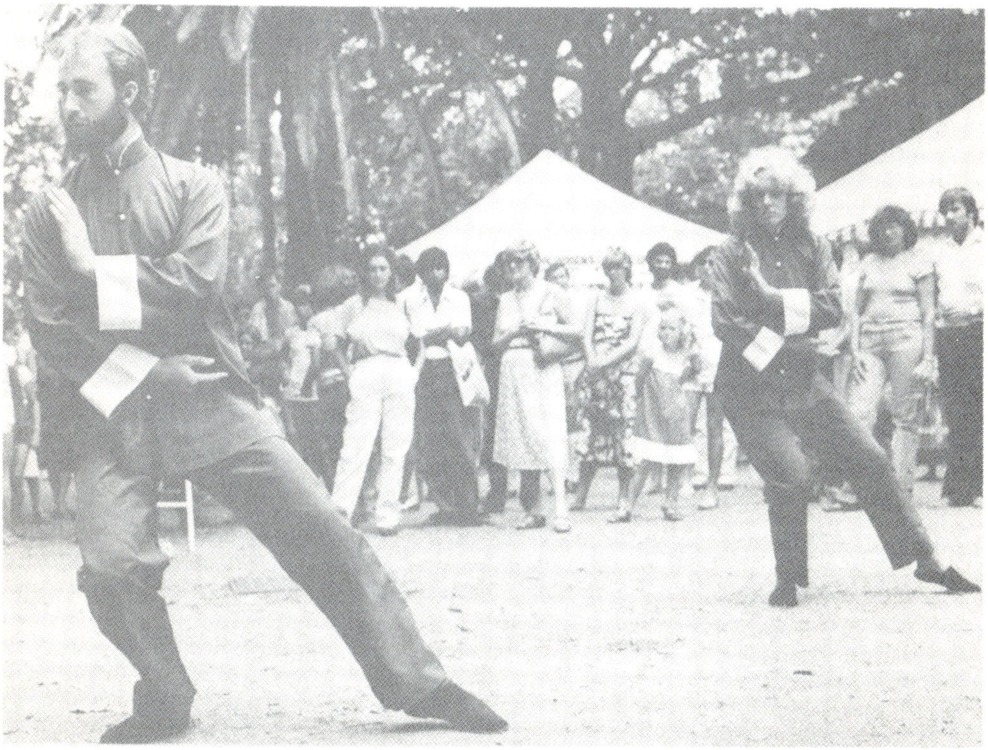

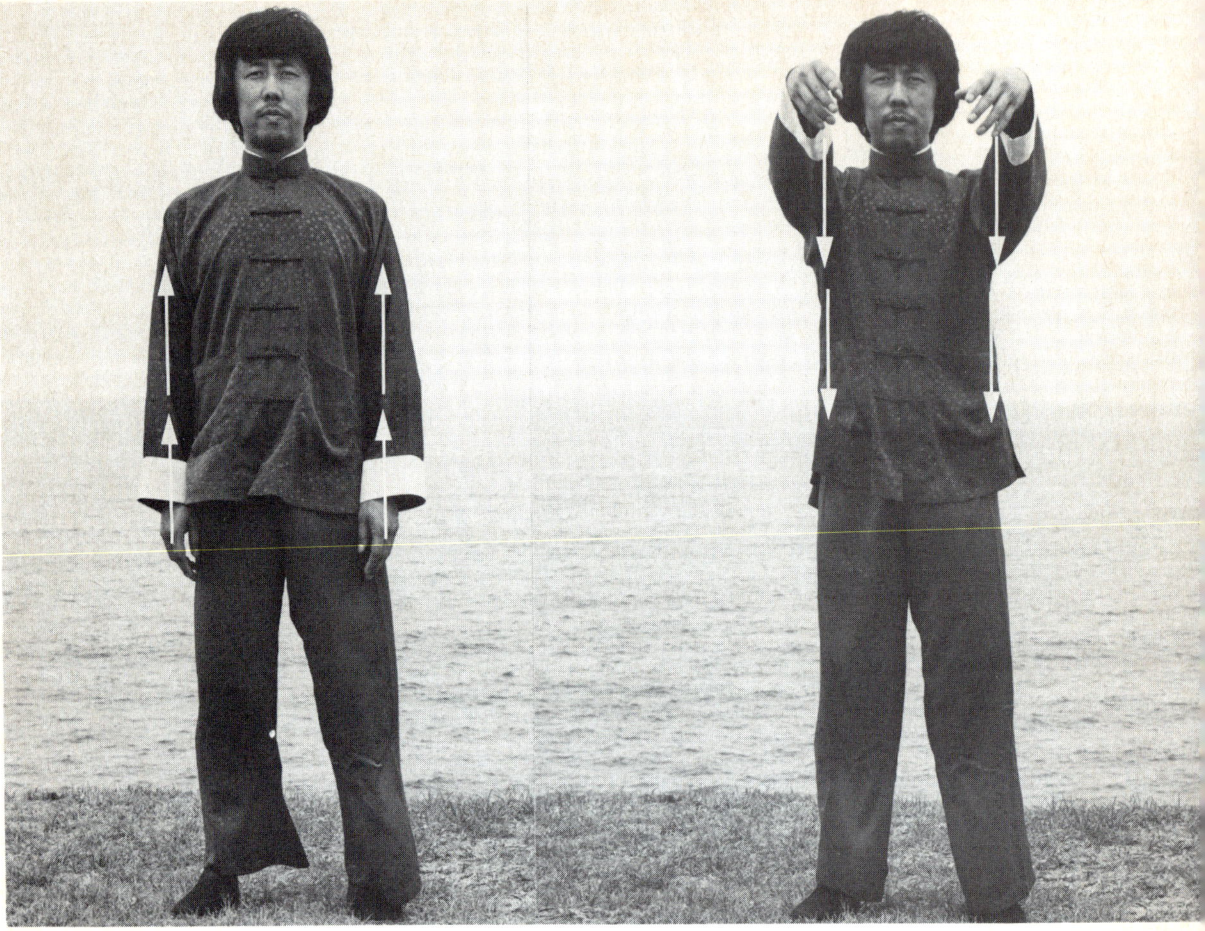

Preparation

Stand with legs about shoulder-width apart, your arms hanging loosely by the side of your body.

Commencement

Raise your arms, palms facing, until they reach eye level. Rotate your wrists inwards so that your palms face the floor. Pull your arms inwards slightly and lower them to the sides of your body.

At the same time bend your knees and lower yourself to a comfortable position, keeping your feet flat on the ground.

When you raise your arms imagine they are being lifted by two balloons attached by string to your wrists — let them float up softly. When you lower your arms push down gently as if you were pushing down a large balloon, and imagine you are lowering yourself into a chair.

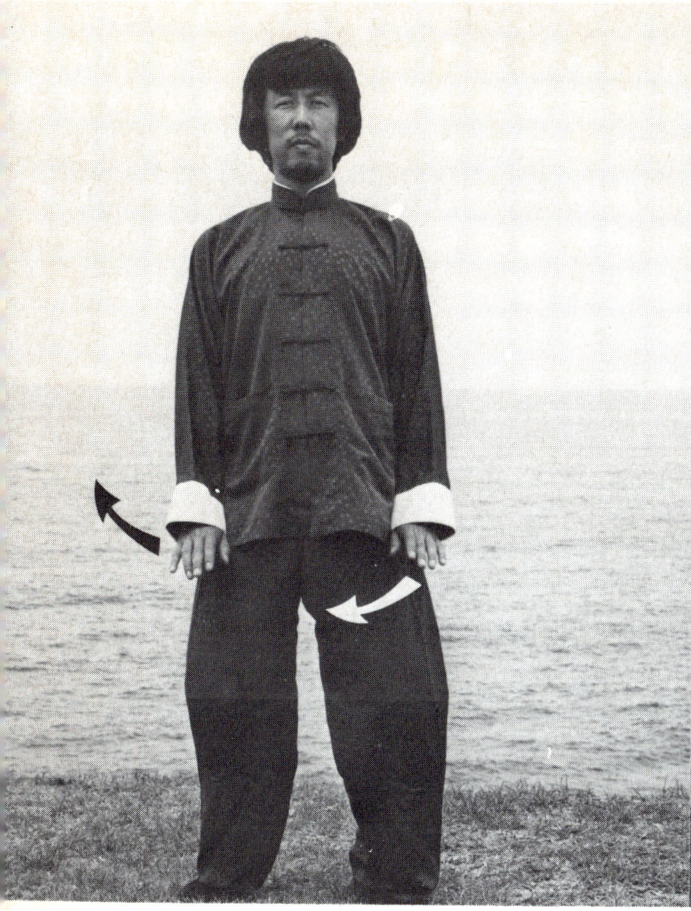

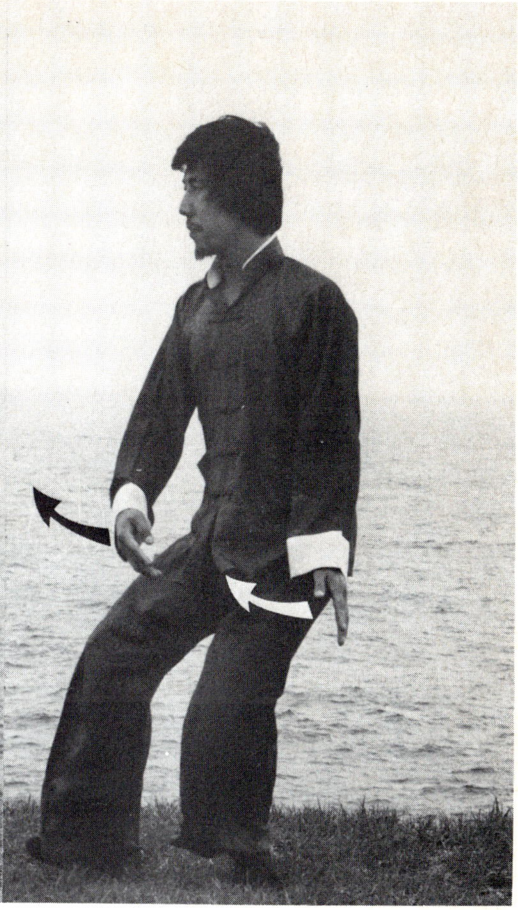

Holding the ball to the right

Footwork

Shift your body weight over to your left leg. Raise the toe of your right foot, leaving the heel on the ground. Pivot on the right heel, turning your body 90 degrees to the right. Lower the toe back to the ground.

Arm movements

Float the right hand up until it reaches eye level, palm facing the floor. Sweep the left arm across to the right side of your body terminating about 1½ feet directly underneath your right hand. The left palm faces upwards.

Co-ordination

Simulate the sitting posture at the end of **Commencement.** Shift your body weight to your left leg. Pivoting on your right heel, rotate your body 90 degrees to the right, then lower your toe back onto the ground. At the same time allow your right hand to float up to eye level as you sweep your left arm across to your right hip. Imagine that your palms are supporting a large ball.

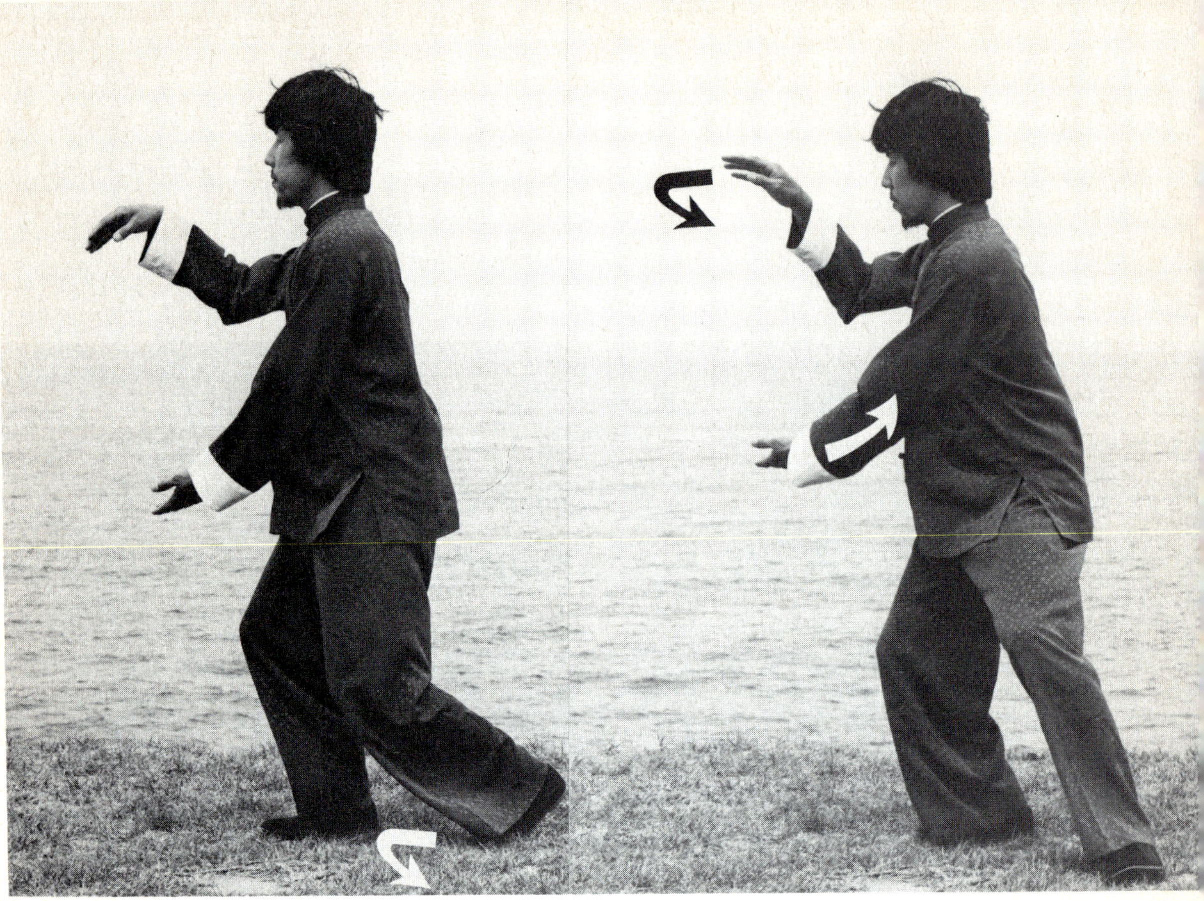

Grasping the bird's tail

Footwork

Transfer your body weight to your right leg. Lift up your left foot and step to the left. Then shift your body weight over to your left leg as you rotate your body back 90 degrees to the left.

Arm movements

Sweep your left hand upwards in an arc across the front of your body, terminating the movement with the wrist directly in front of your chest, palm facing inwards. Your right hand sweeps down to your right hip. 70% of your body weight should be carried by your left leg and 30% by the right leg.

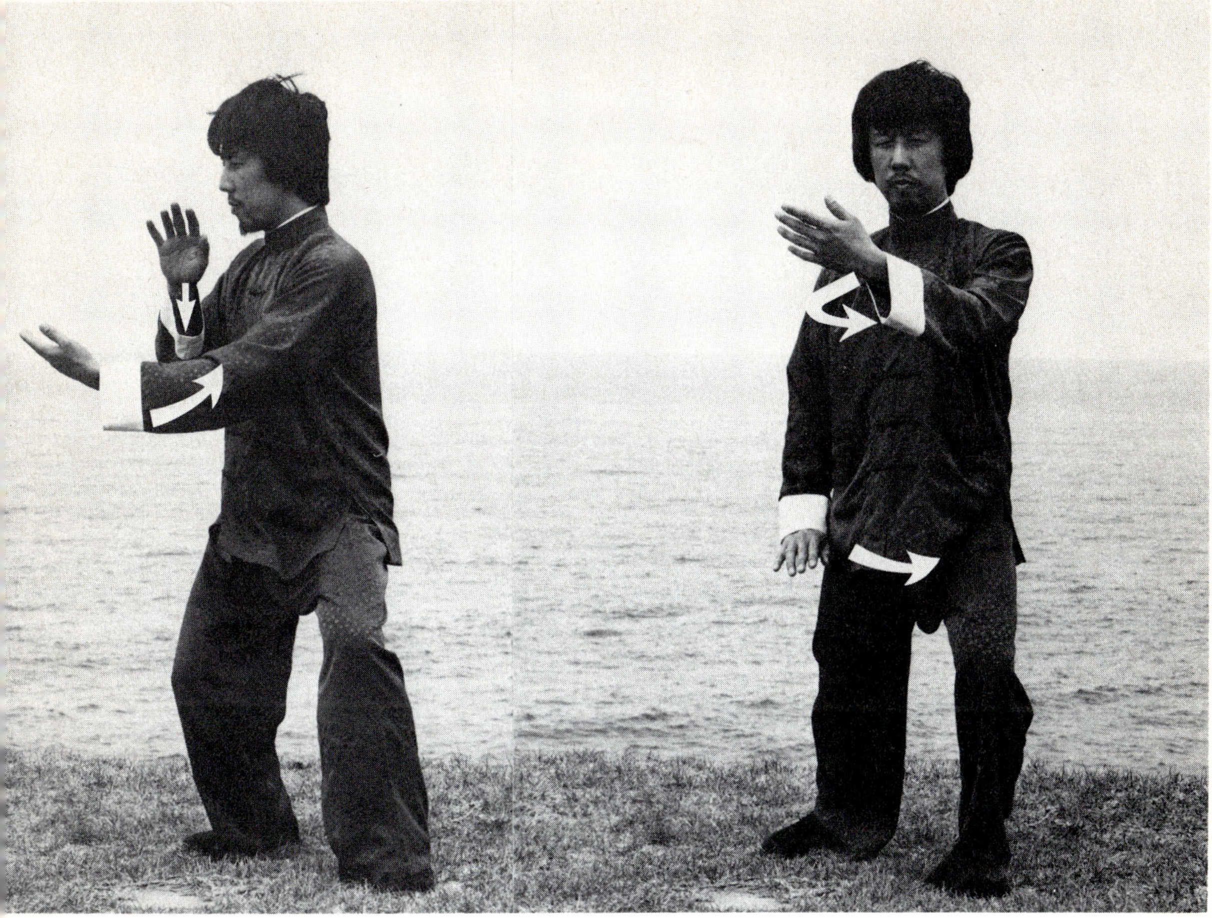

Co-ordination

From the posture of **Holding the ball to the right** shift your weight to the right leg and step to the left with your left foot. Now, imagine there is a bird standing on your left wrist and your right palm is poised over its head. As you rotate your body 90 degrees to the left and shift your body weight forward to the left leg, sweep your right palm downwards as if you were stroking the bird down to the end of its tail. At the same time your left arm sweeps across the body and upwards, as if releasing the bird into flight.

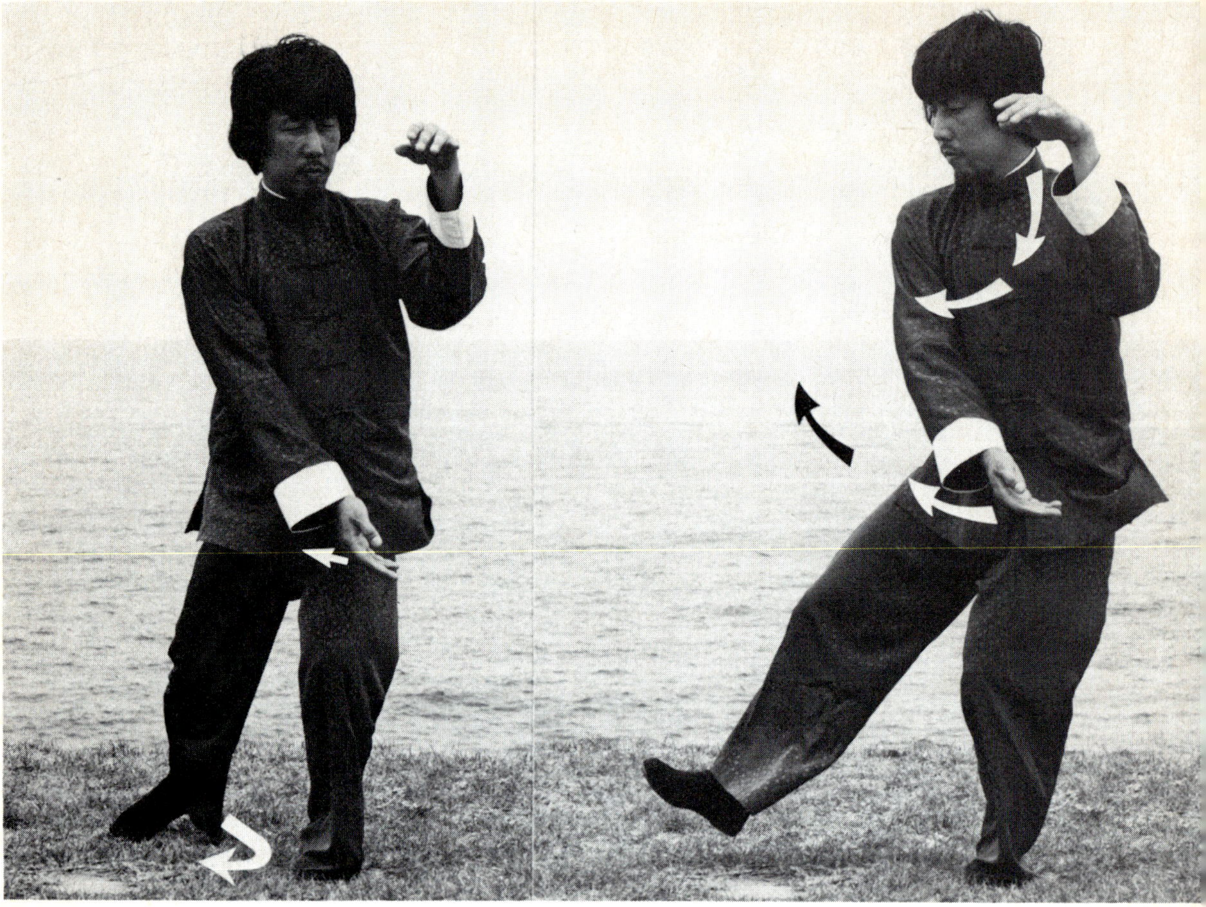

Holding the ball to the left

From **Grasping the bird's tail** rotate your left wrist so that the palm faces the ground. At the same time sweep your right hand across to the left side of your body, terminating 1½ feet directly underneath your left hand, with your right palm facing up. Imagine your hands are supporting a large ball.

Ward off

Footwork

With your weight on your left leg, lift your right foot, bring it in to your left foot and step to the right in a circular movement. Shift your weight to the right leg as you rotate your body 90 degrees to the right. 70% of your body weight should be carried by your right leg and 30% by your left leg.

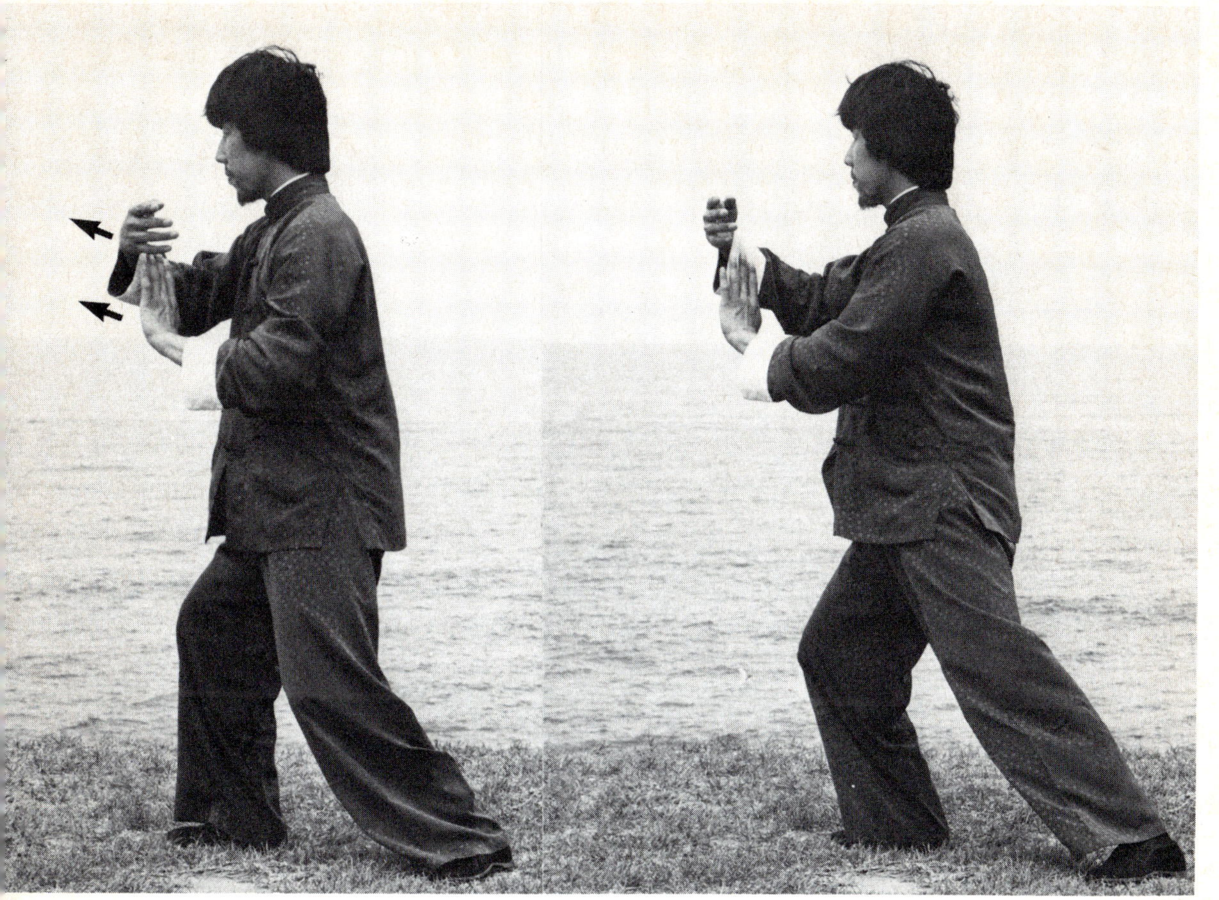

Arm movements

Sweep your right hand upwards in an arc to the front of your body, palm facing you. Push forward and down with your left palm, terminating the movement just underneath your right wrist.

Co-ordination

From **Holding the ball to the left** step to the right with your right foot. Turn your body 90 degrees to the right as you shift your body weight over to your right foot. As you turn your body, sweep your right hand upwards and your left hand forwards to just underneath your right wrist.

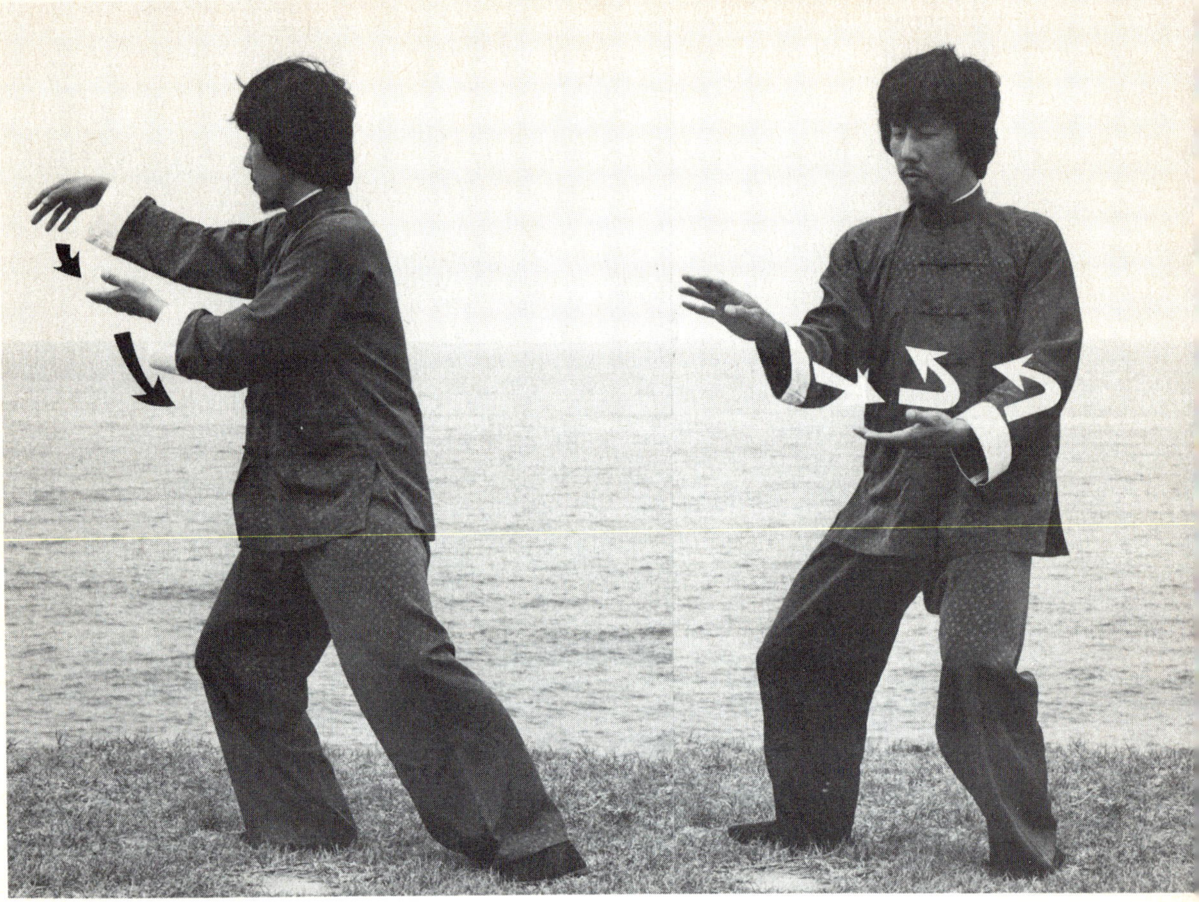

Pull Back

Footwork

Twist your body slightly to the left as you shift your weight back to your left leg.

Arm movements

Turn your wrists so that your right palm faces downwards and your left palm faces up. Contract both arms slightly inwards and let the twisting of your body pull your arms back.

Co-ordination

From **Ward off** turn your wrists so that the right palm faces down and the left palm faces up. Imagine that you are pulling something towards you as you contract your arms, twist your body to the left and shift your weight to your left leg, all in one smooth movement.

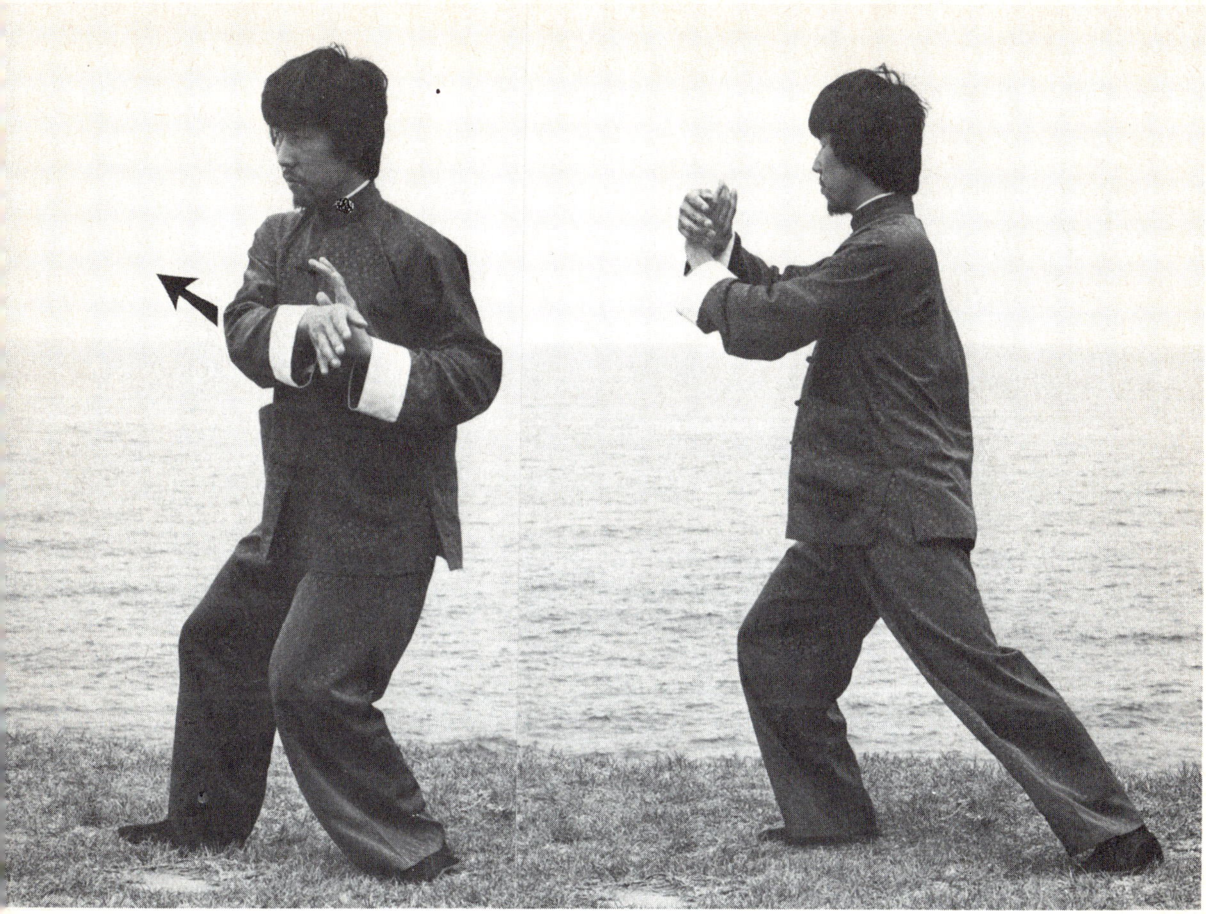

Press forward

Footwork

Twist your body back to the right and transfer your weight to the right leg.

Arm movements

Turn your right palm to face you, place your left palm on the right wrist. Extend your left arm to press out onto your right wrist and push it forward.

Co-ordination

From **Pull Back** as you twist your body back to the right, turn your right palm inwards and place your left palm on your right wrist. As you transfer your body weight to the right press outwards onto your right wrist with your left palm.

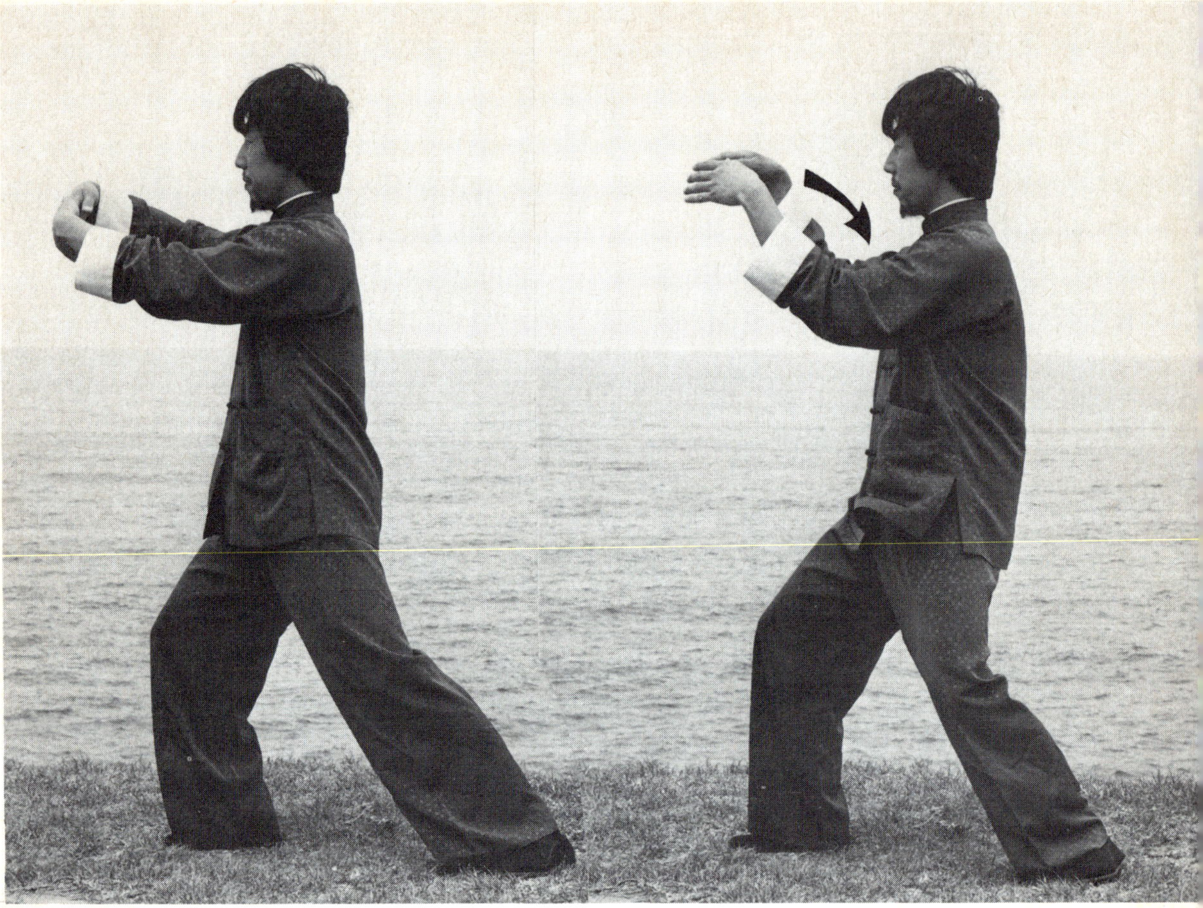

Extend arms to push

Footwork

Transfer your weight first back to the left leg, and then forwards again to the right.

Arm movements

Separate your hands and pull them in towards your body in a circle. Then extend both arms to push.

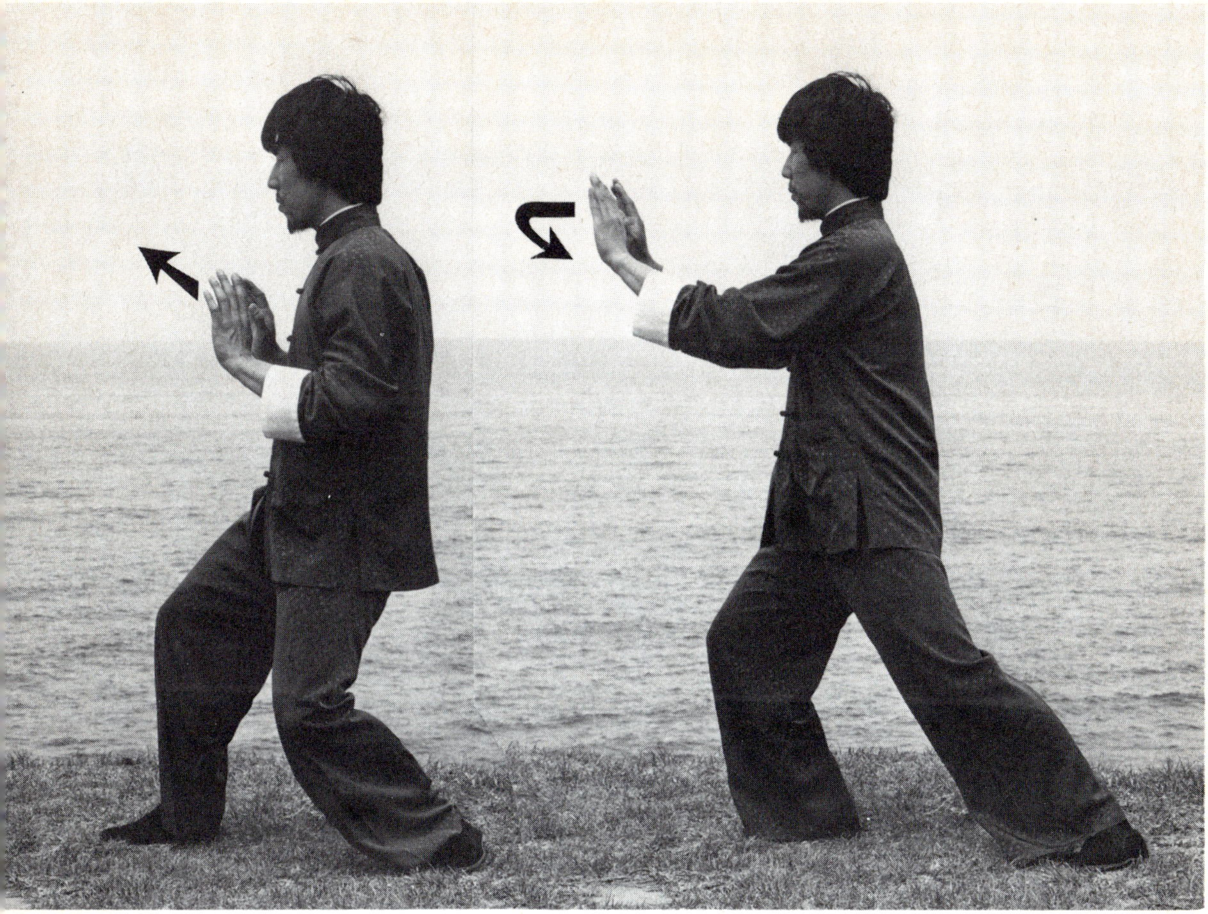

Co-ordination

From **Press forward** part your hands and contract your arms inwards as you shift your body weight backwards to your left leg. Then extend your arms as if to shut a door, at the same time shifting your weight forward to the right leg.

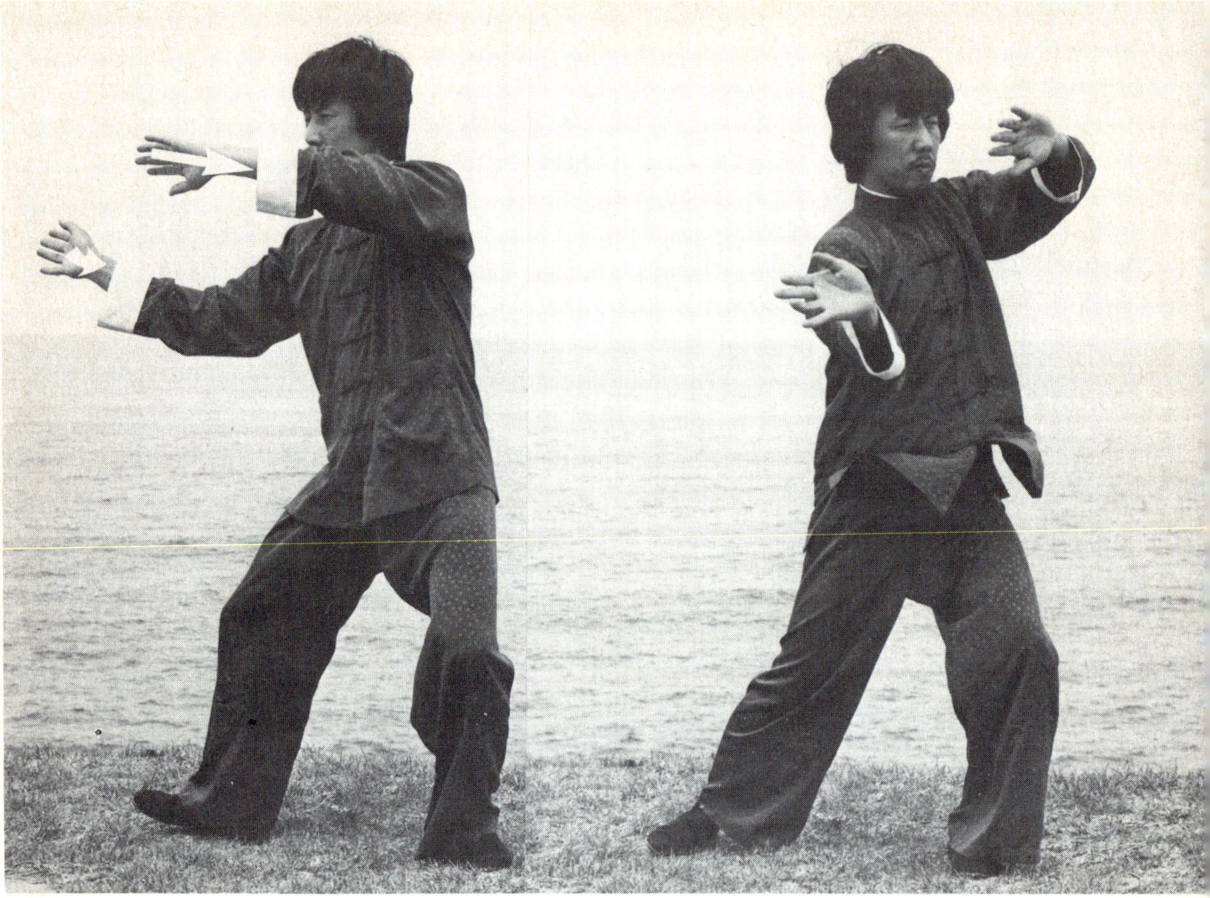

Single whip A

Footwork

Shift your weight back to the left leg, lift your right toe. Pivot on your right heel and turn your body 180 degrees to the left.

Arm movements

With both palms facing outwards, contract your arms slightly and let your body pull your arms around.

Co-ordination

From **Extend arms to push** shift your weight to the left leg. Pivoting on your right heel turn your body 180 degrees to the left, contracting your arms slightly so that they sweep round with your body, palms facing out.

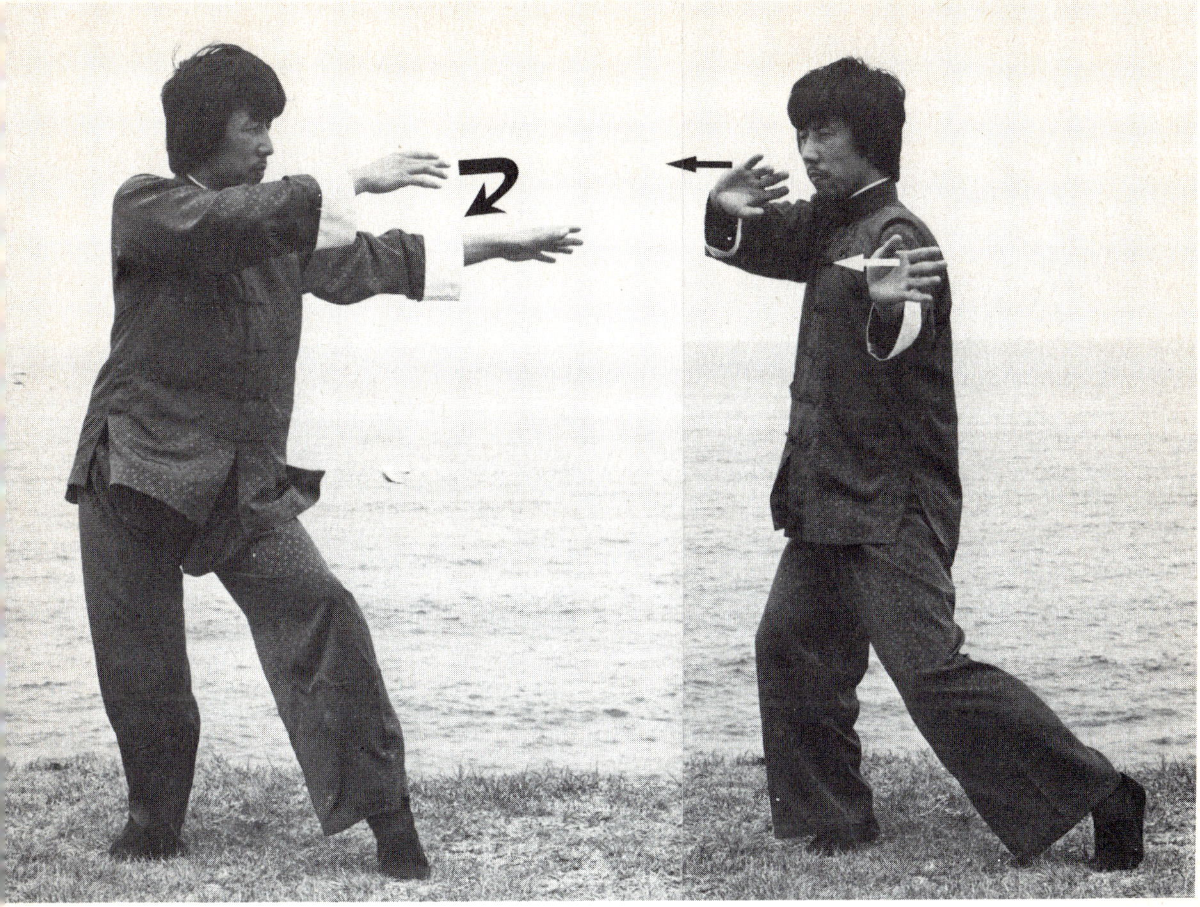

Single whip B

Footwork

Shift your weight to the right leg. Raise your left heel so that you pivot on your left toe. Turn your body 180 degrees back to the right.

Arm movements

With both palms still facing outwards, contract your arms slightly.

Co-ordination

From **Single whip A** shift your weight to the right leg and pivoting on the left toe, spin 180 degrees back to the right. Contract your arms slightly as you turn so that your body pulls your arms around with it.

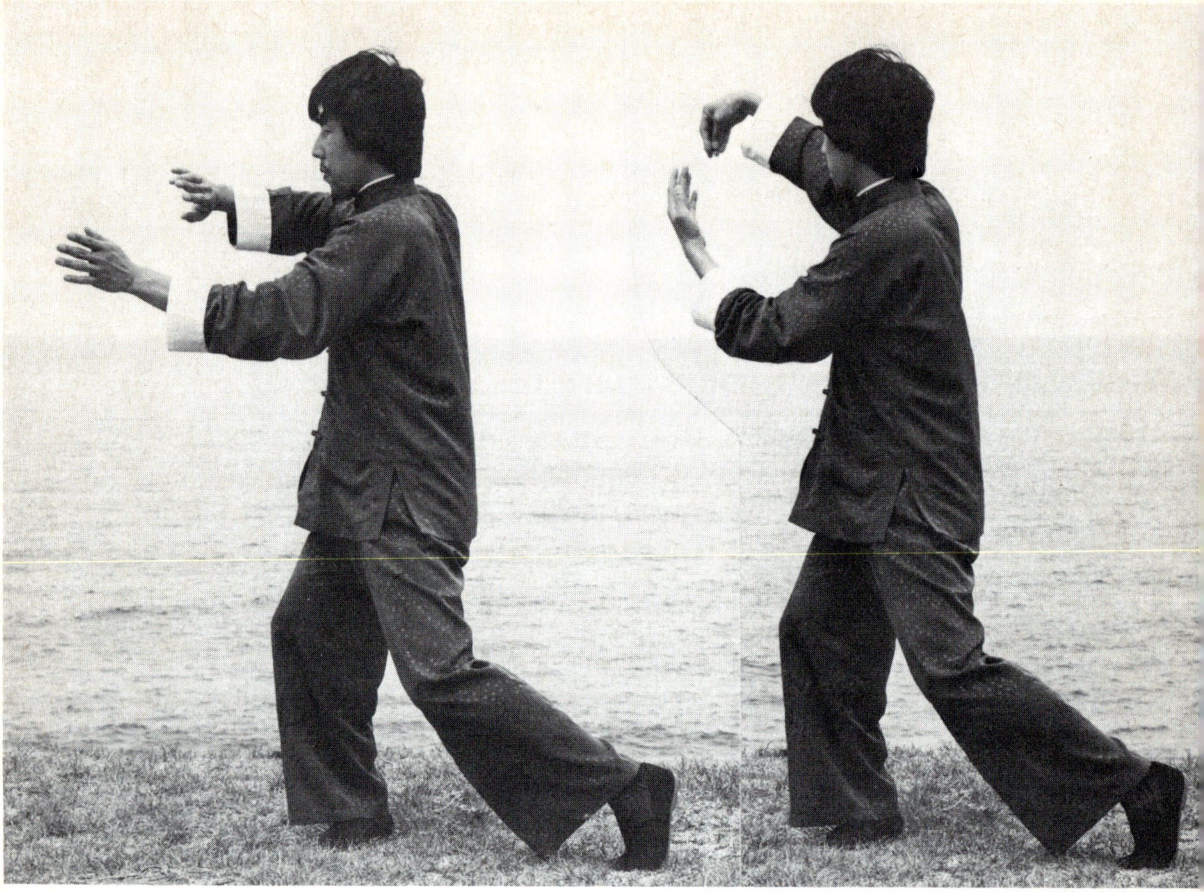

Single whip C

Footwork

Maintain the weight on your right leg. Pivot on your left toe, turning the body 180 degrees to the left again. Step to the left with your left foot and transfer the weight forward to the left leg, placing your foot flat on the ground.

Arm movements

Make a hook with your right hand and turn your left palm in to face you, as if you were holding a mirror. At the end of the 180 degree spin, turn your left palm outwards and extend your left arm to push.

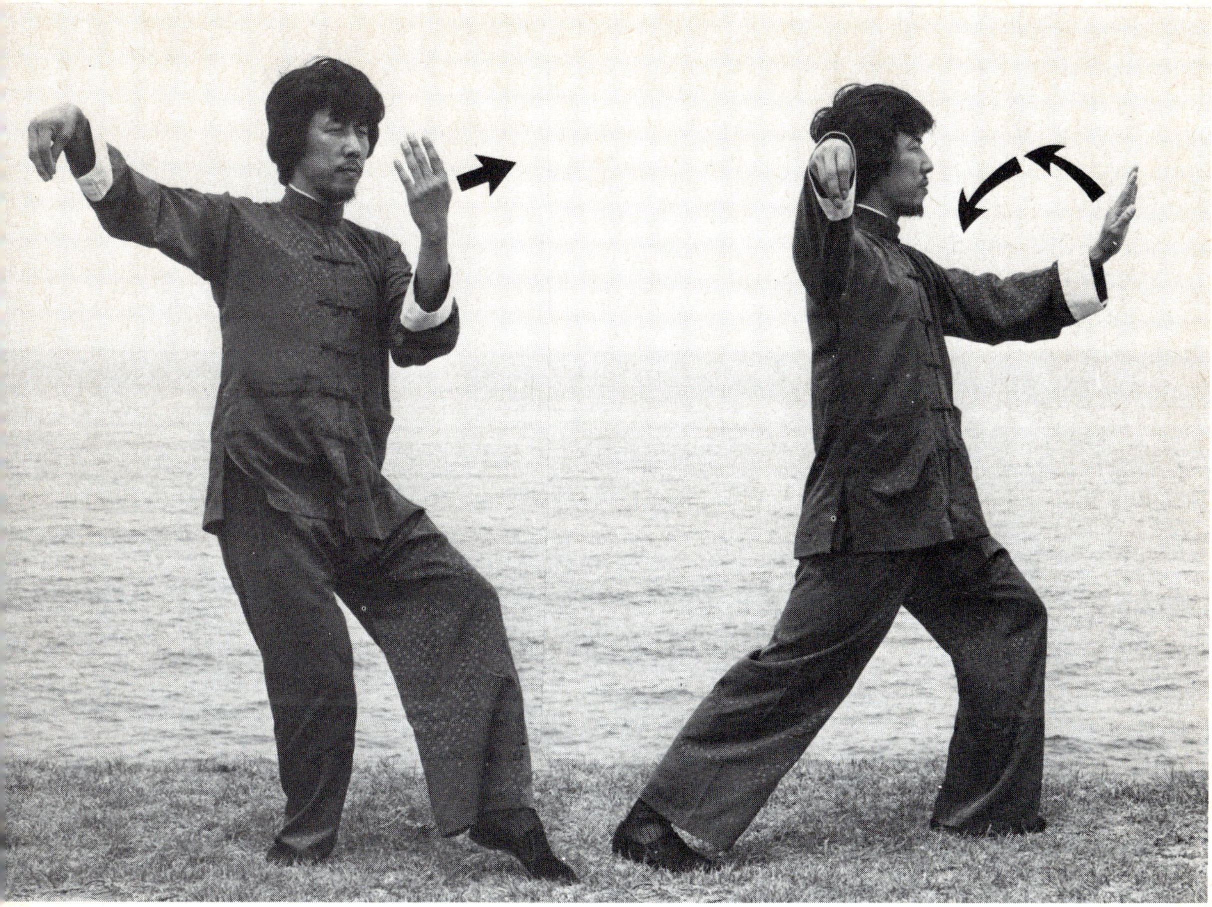

Co-ordination

From **Single whip B** make a hook with your right hand and turn your left palm to face you. With your body weight still on your right leg, and pivoting on your left toe, spin your body 180 degrees to the left. Then step to the left with your left foot and turn your left palm outwards. As you shift your body weight forward to your left leg, extend your left arm to push outwards.

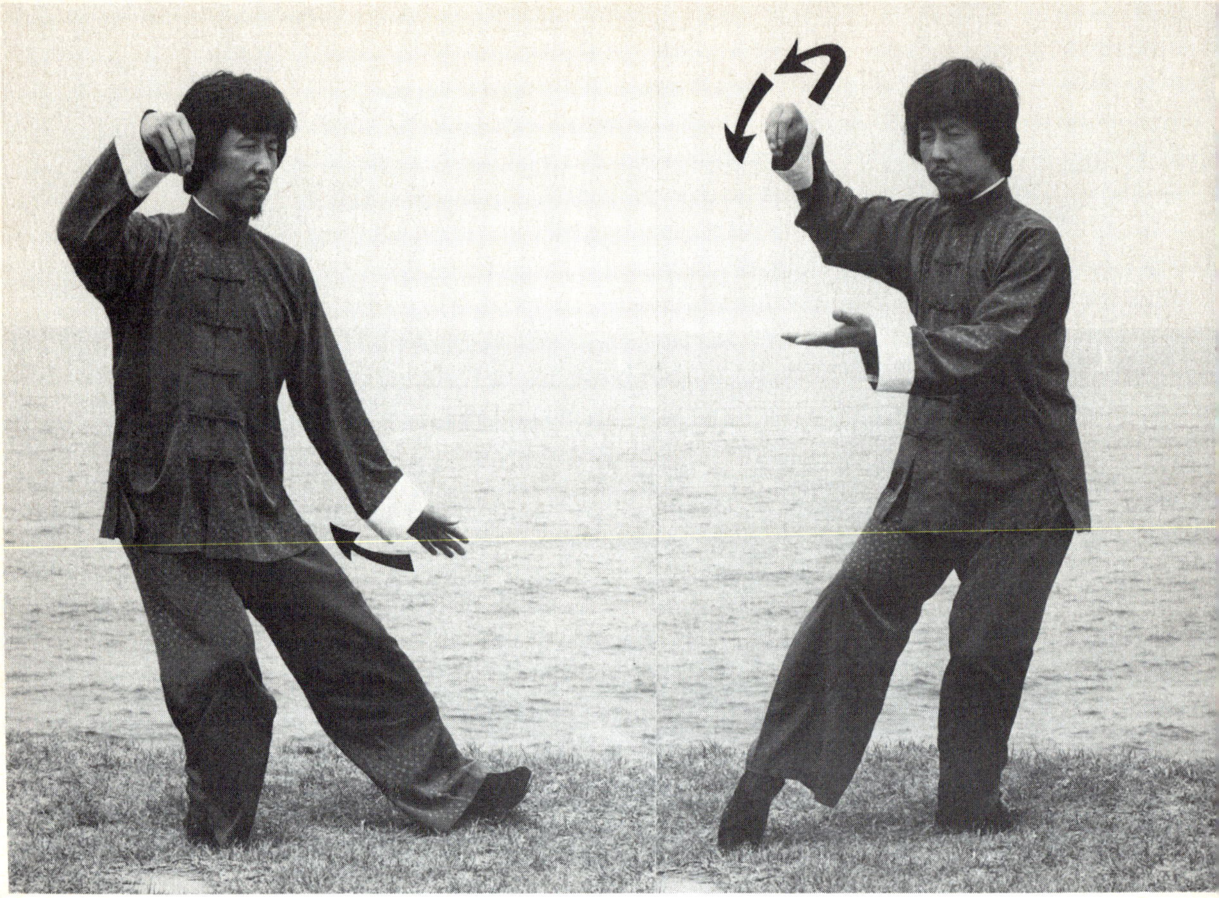

Play guitar

Footwork

Shift your weight back to the right leg. Lift your left toe and pivoting on your left heel, rotate your body 90 degrees to the right. Place your left foot flat on the ground and transfer your weight to the left leg. Lift up your right foot and place it in front with only the heel touching the ground and the weight on the left leg.

Arm movements

Draw your left arm to the back and sweep it round to the front in a big circular anti-clockwise movement. Your hand will finish just in front of your chest. Then draw your right arm to the back in a big circular clockwise sweep. Your right hand will finish to the front of your chest and above the left, palms facing.

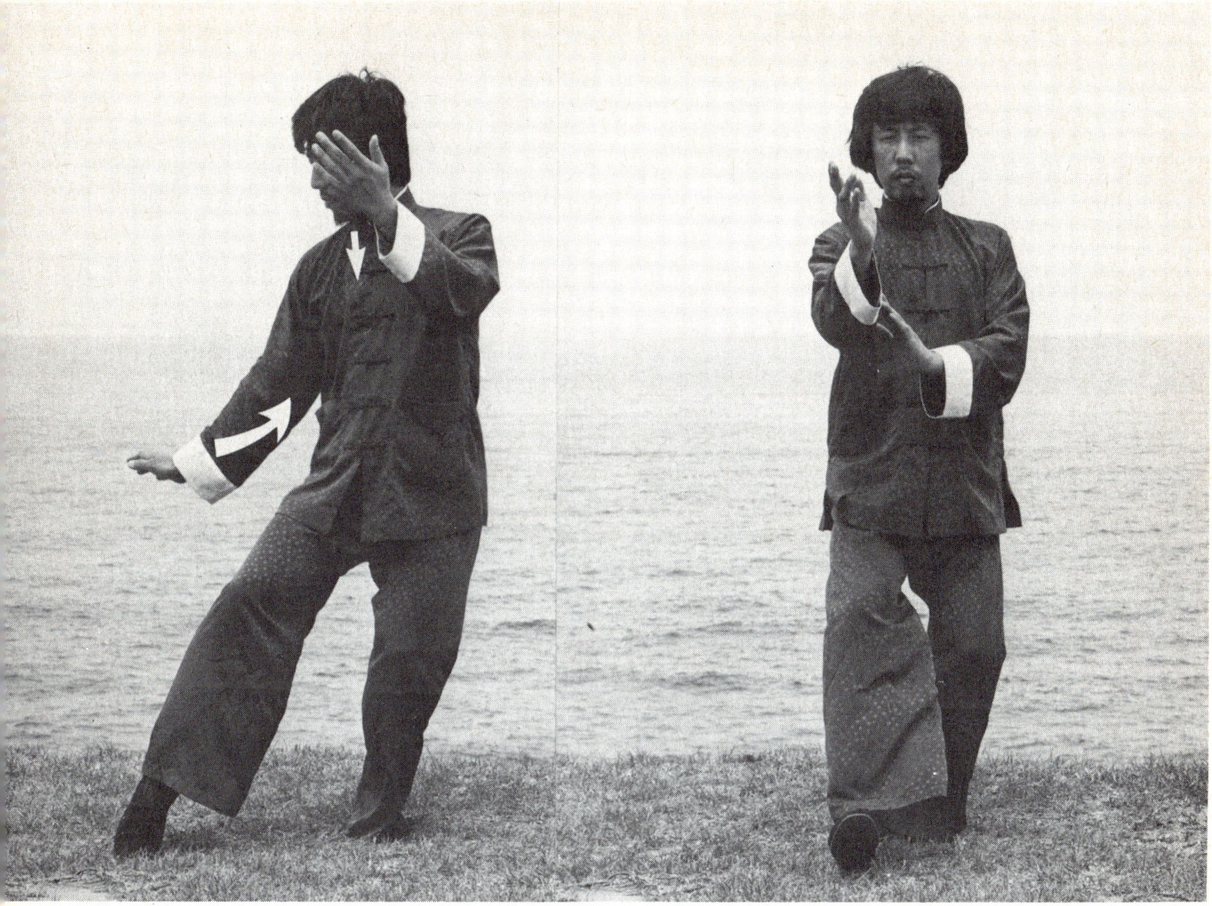

Co-ordination

From **Single whip C** shift your body weight back to the right leg. Draw your left arm back in a sweep as you pivot on your left heel and rotate your body 90 degrees to the right. Transfer your weight to the left leg. Now draw your right arm back to do a clockwise sweep to the front of your chest, at the same time lifting your right foot and placing it down in front of you with only the right heel touching the ground.

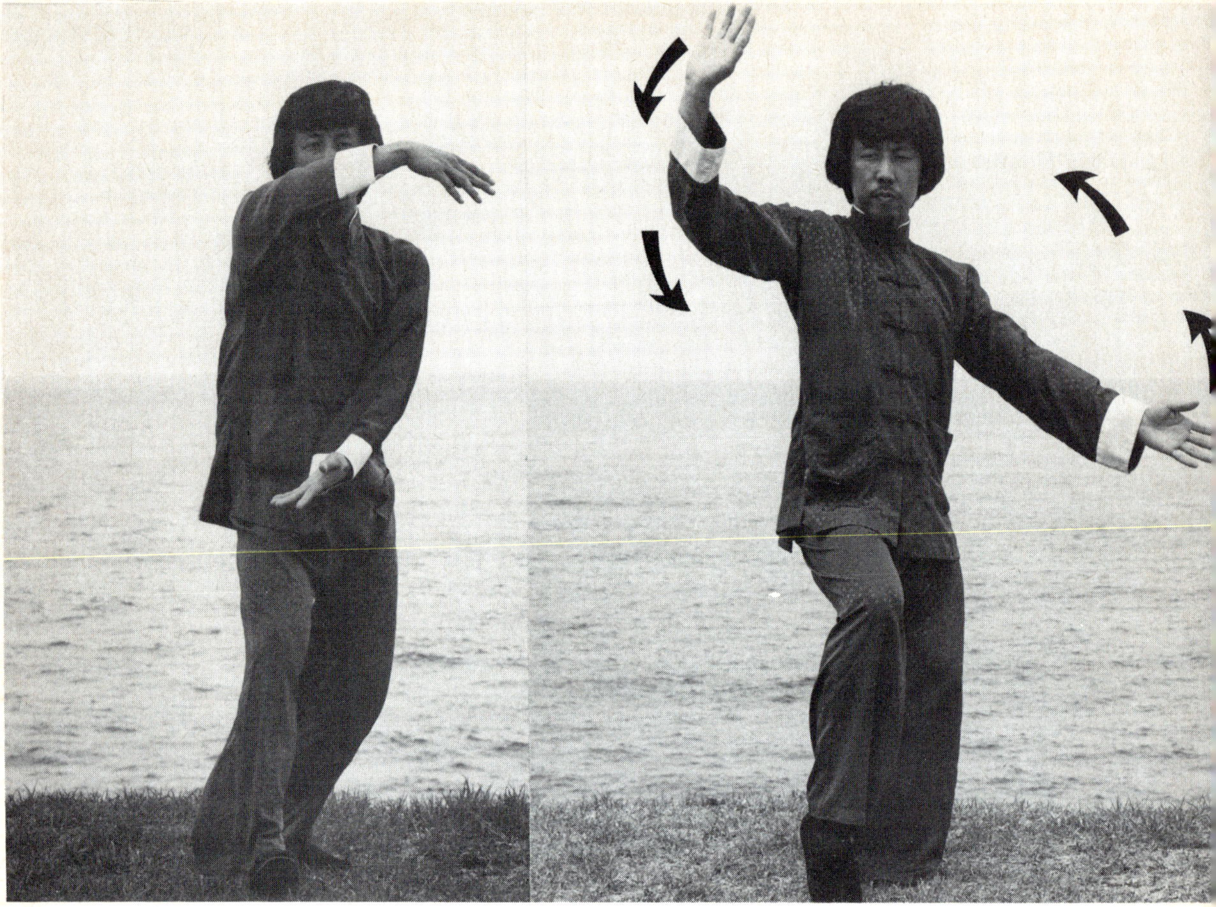

Shoulder stroke

Footwork

Draw your right foot in to pivot on your right toe momentarily. Step forward with your right foot to the front. Shift your body weight forward to your right leg.

Arm movements

Sweep your right arm up and your left arm down as though you were turning a car steering wheel to the right. Your left hand comes to rest just underneath your chin, palm facing the front. Your right arm finishes by the side of your left hip.

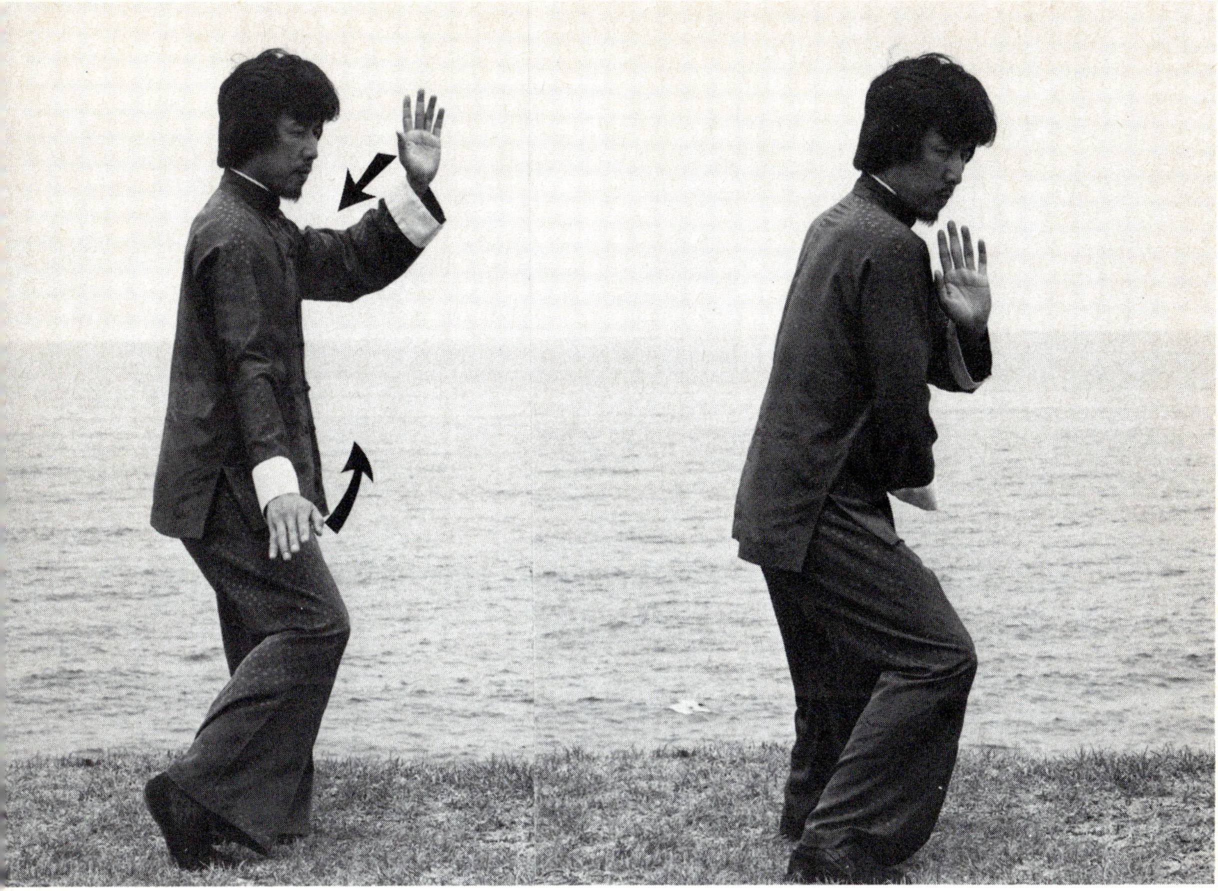

Co-ordination

From **Play guitar** draw your right foot in to pivot on the toe, as you spin your arms in a clockwise circle. Terminate the arm movements with the left hand under your chin, and the right hand by your left hip. Step forward with your right foot and push forward to ram with your right shoulder.

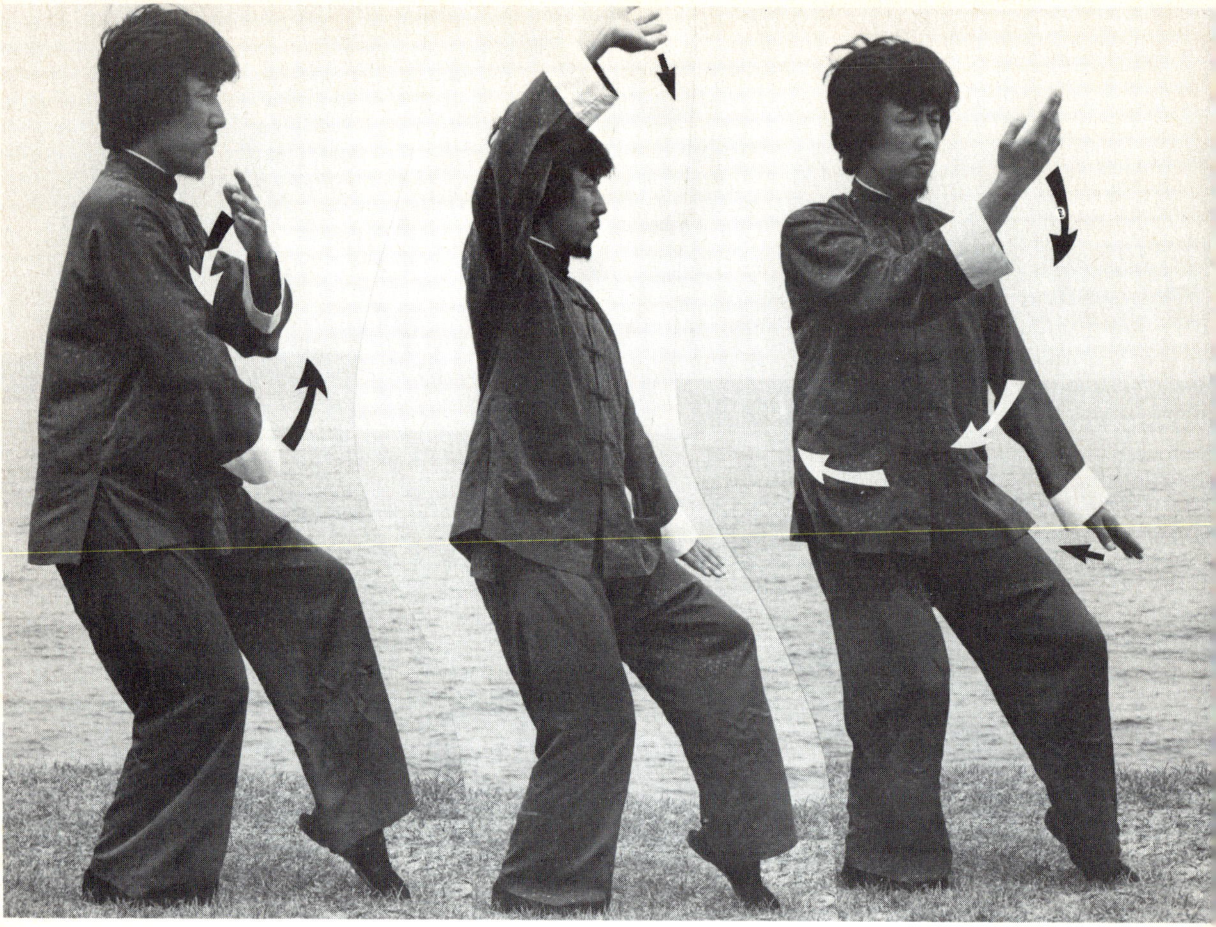

White crane spreads wings

Footwork

Maintaining your weight on your right leg, bring your left foot forward, coming to rest on your left toe.

Arm movements

Turn your head to face the front. Push your left hand down to your left hip. Raise your right hand to chest level, rotate palm outwards and push up.

Co-ordination

From **Shoulder stroke** turn your head 90 degrees to the left, as you sweep your left foot forward to balance on your left toe. At the same time separate both arms, right hand sweeping up to your head and left hand sweeping down to your left hip.

Brush knee

Arm movements

Rotate your right wrist to turn your right palm inwards to face you. Then allow your right arm to sink downwards, circling it to the

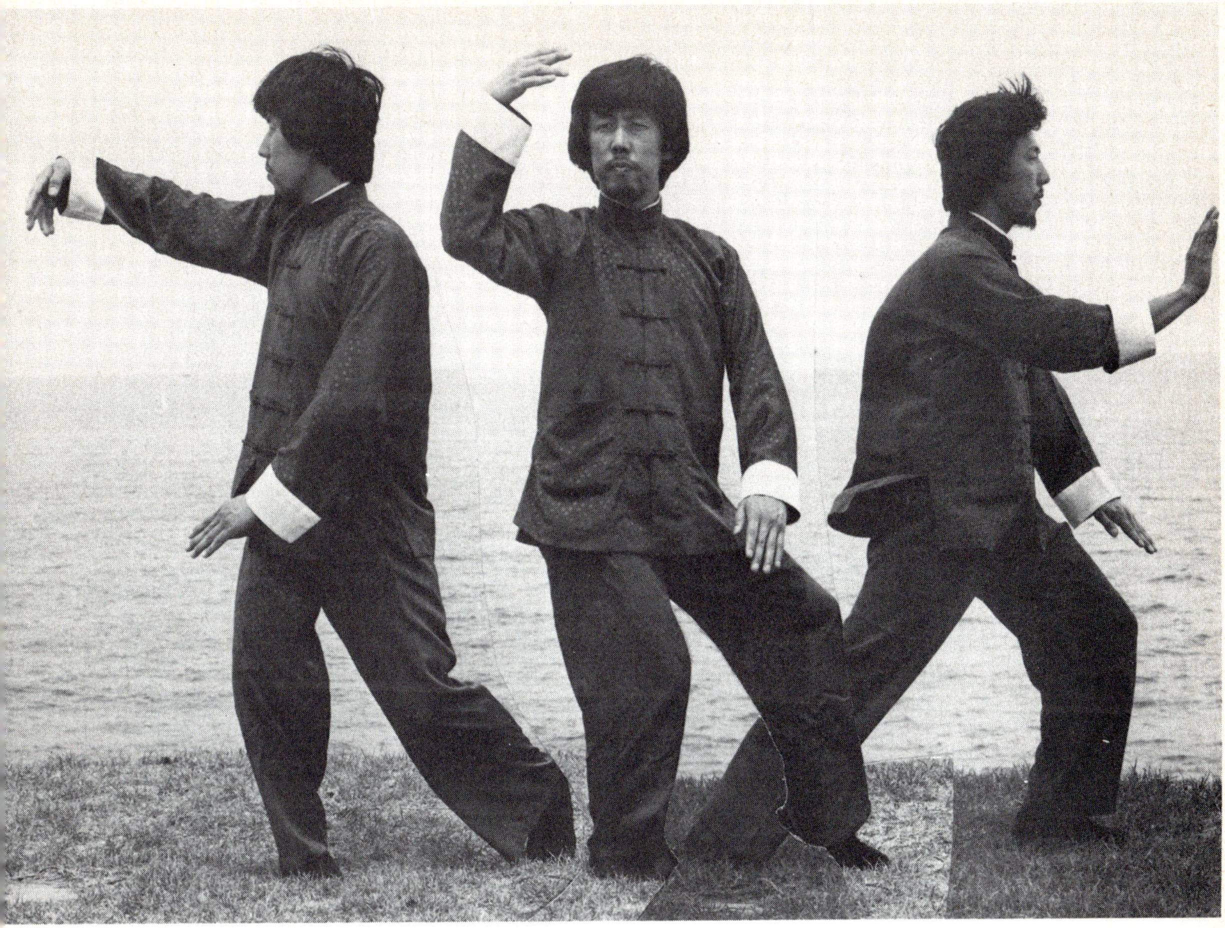

back, to come up over your head. The turning of your body in turn draws your left arm upwards in a partial sweeping motion. Turning your body back to the left, let your left hand brush past your left knee, then press forward with the right palm.

Footwork

Turn your head to follow the backward flow of your right arm. Then turn your body back to the left and step to the left with your left foot. Shift your body weight forward to the left leg.

Co-ordination

From the **White crane** turn your right palm in to face you and allow your right arm to sweep down to the back, then up over your head. Simultaneously, roll your body and head to follow the sweep, and in turn, draw your left arm upwards. Then step to the left with your left foot, and as you brush your left palm over your left knee, press forward with your right plam and shift your body weight forward to your left leg.

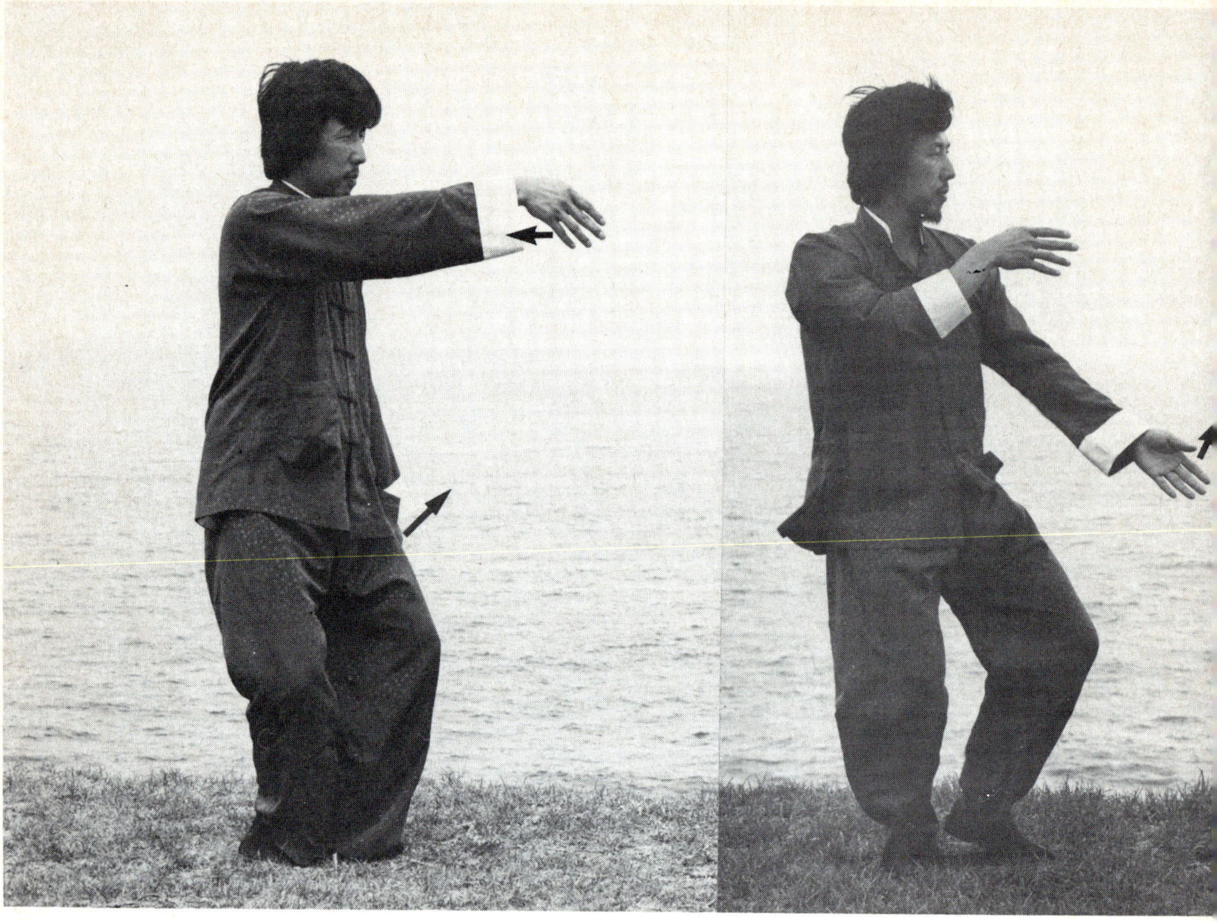

Play guitar

Footwork

Take a step forward with your right foot and place it down close behind your left foot. Pass your body weight over to your right leg so that you can lift up your left foot, and then place your left foot down in front with only the heel touching the ground.

Arm movements

Drop your right wrist so your fingers point downwards. Draw your right arm in close to your chest, while the left arm sweeps up to the front.

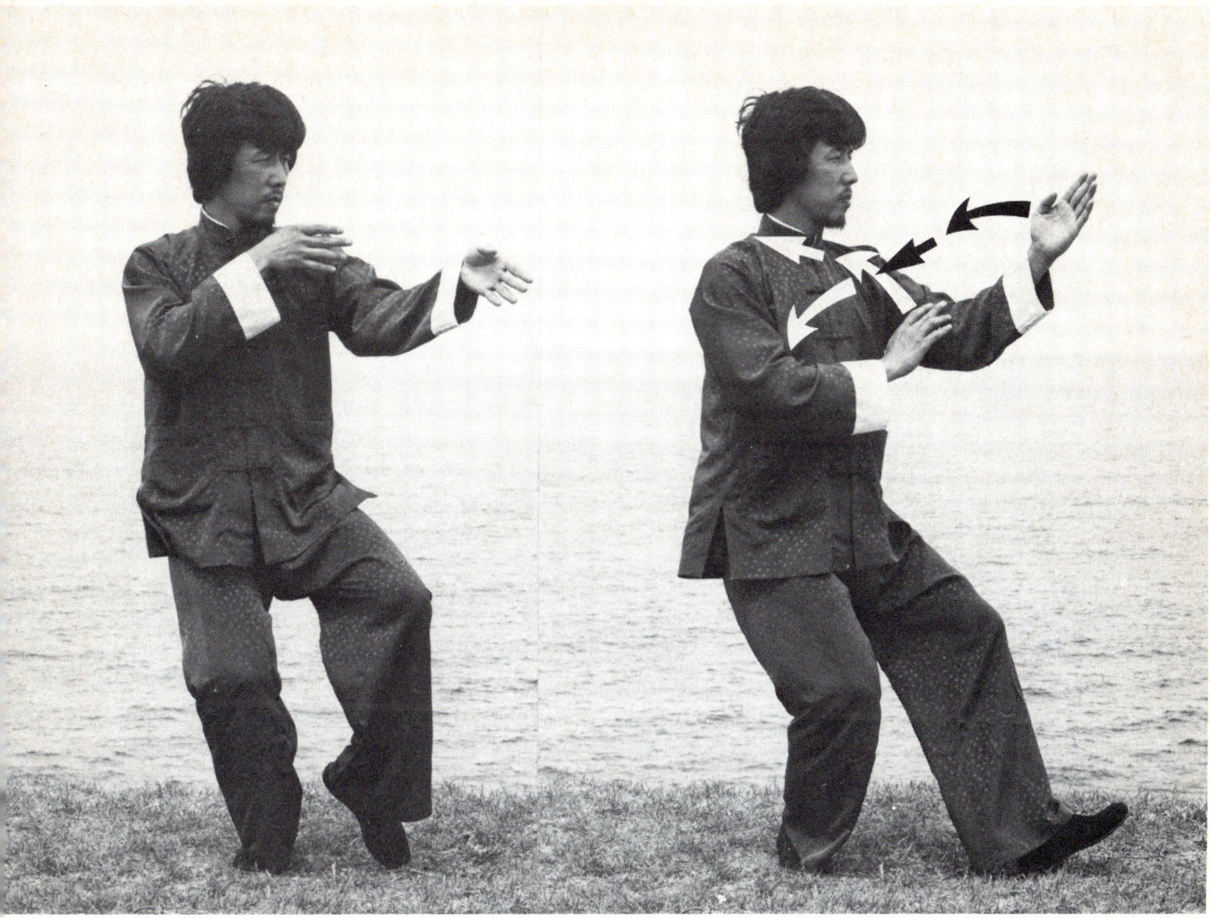

Co-ordination

From **Brush knee** step forward with your right foot, placing it close behind your left foot. As you transfer your body weight over to your right foot, draw your right arm in and place it near your chest. Lift up your left foot and pivot your left heel in front of your body as you sweep your left arm up to the front. This posture is the mirror image of the first **Play guitar.**

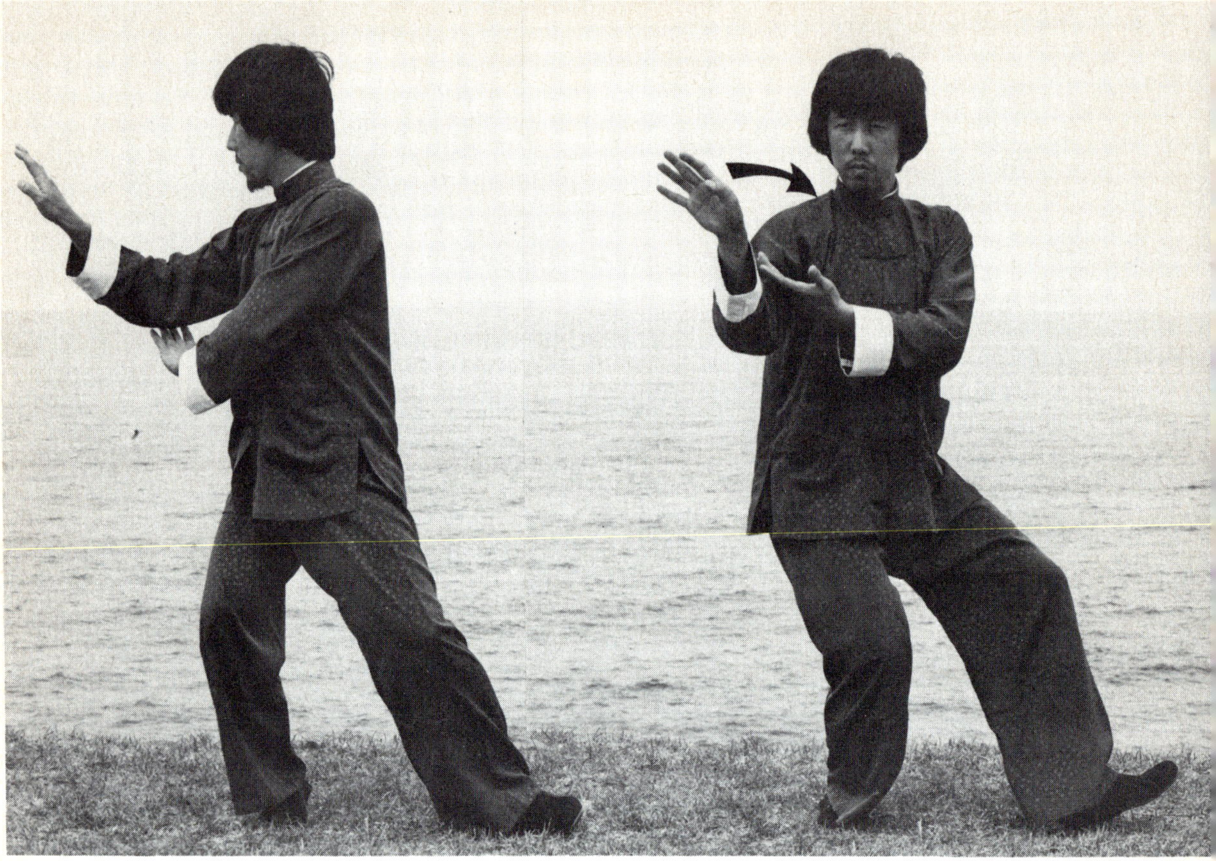

Slant flying

Footwork

Maintaining your weight on the right foot, and pivoting on your left heel, rotate your body 180 degrees to the right. Still maintaining your weight on the right foot, pivot back on your left heel 180 degrees to the left. Step to the left with your left foot. Shift your body weight to the left leg.

Arm movements

As you rotate your body 180 degrees to the right, sweep your left hand down to your right hip, and right hand up to eye level. As you rotate back to the left, separate your arms in opposite directions, your left palm sweeping upwards to the left, your right palm sweeping downwards to the right.

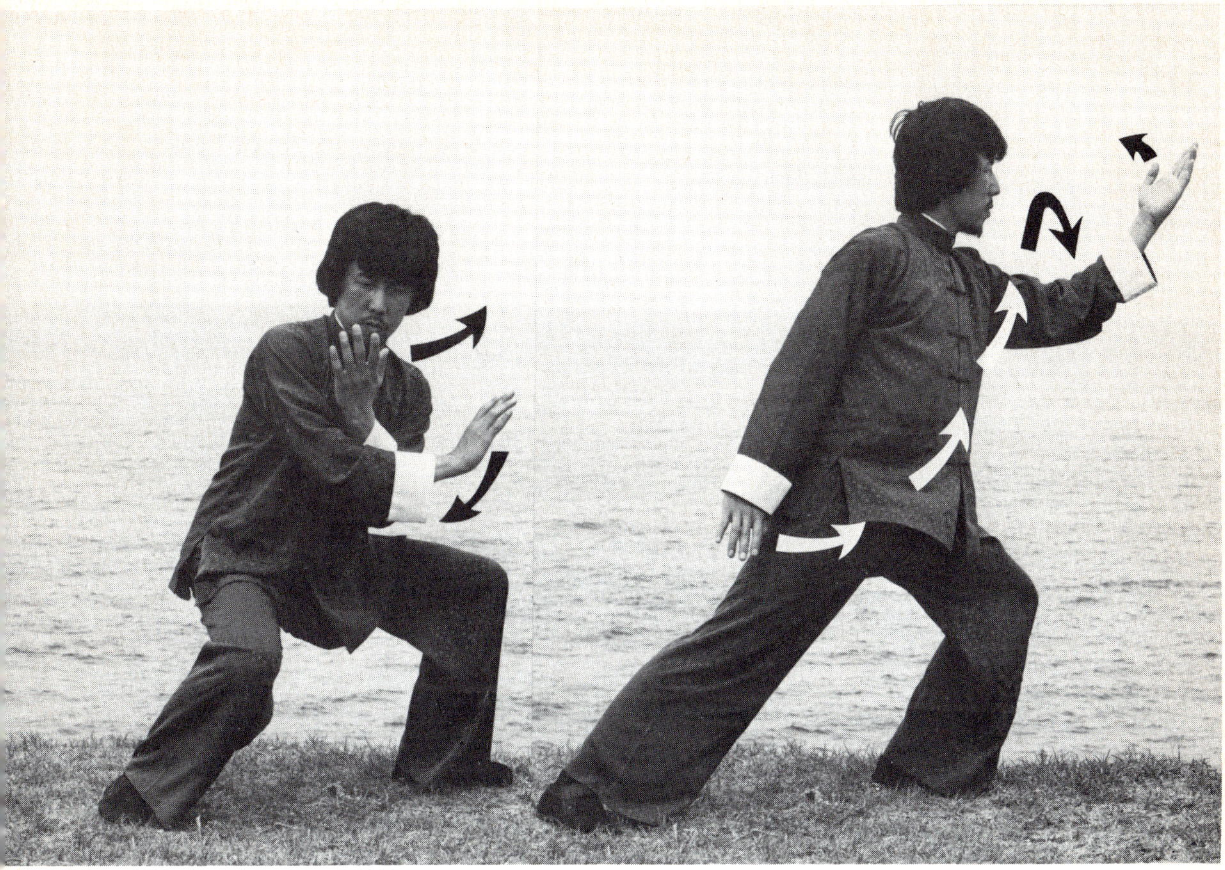

Co-ordination

Starting from **Play guitar** keep your weight on the right foot and pivot on the left heel. Rotate your body 180 degrees to the right, and at the same time, sweep your left hand down to your right hip, and right hand up to eye level. Rotate your body 180 degrees to the left, and step to the left with your left foot. As you shift your body weight forward to your left leg, sweep your left palm upwards to the left, and right palm downwards to the right.

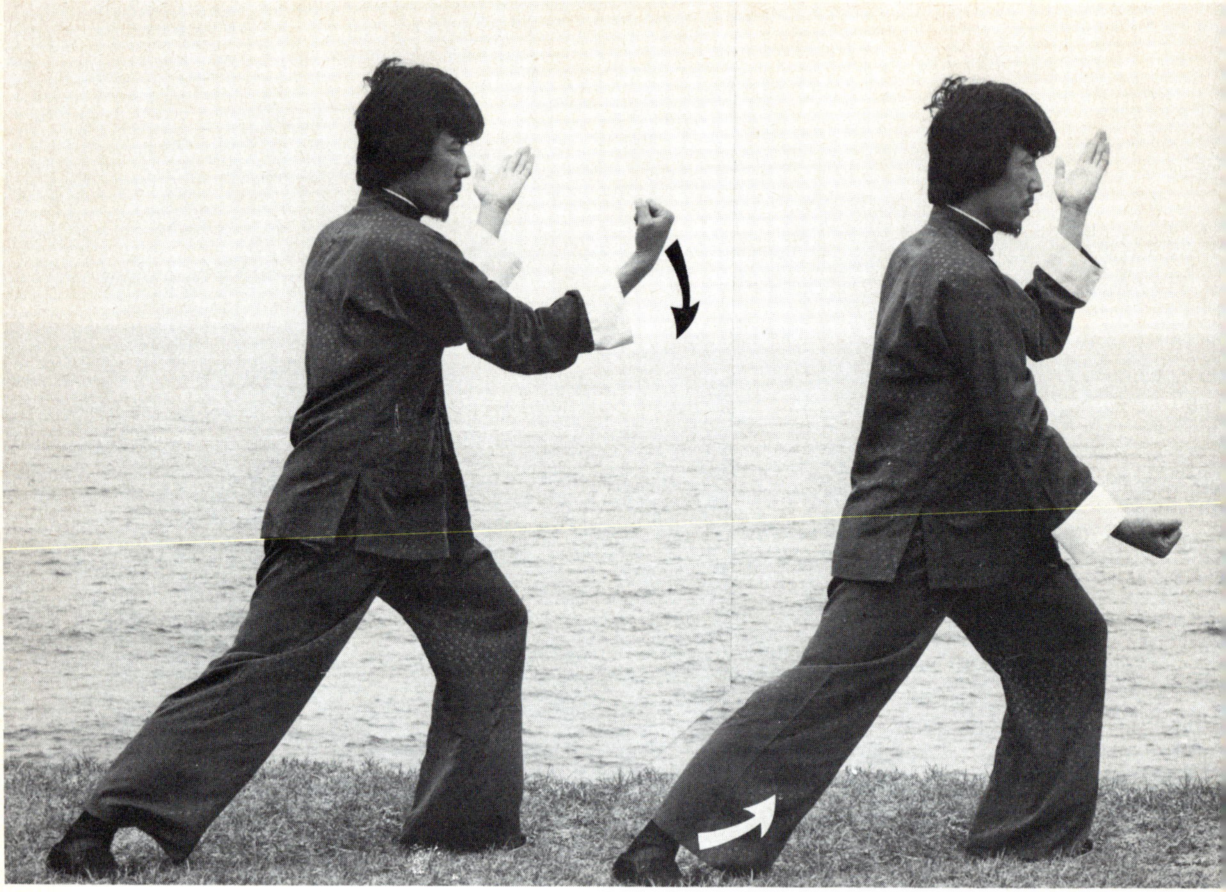

Cross deflection

Make a fist with your right hand, and do a back-handed sweep from your right hip, across the front of your body, up to the left side of your head, and then down the front to finish between your legs.

Kick and thrust

Footwork

Transfer all your body weight to the left leg. Lift up your right knee and extend your right leg to kick.

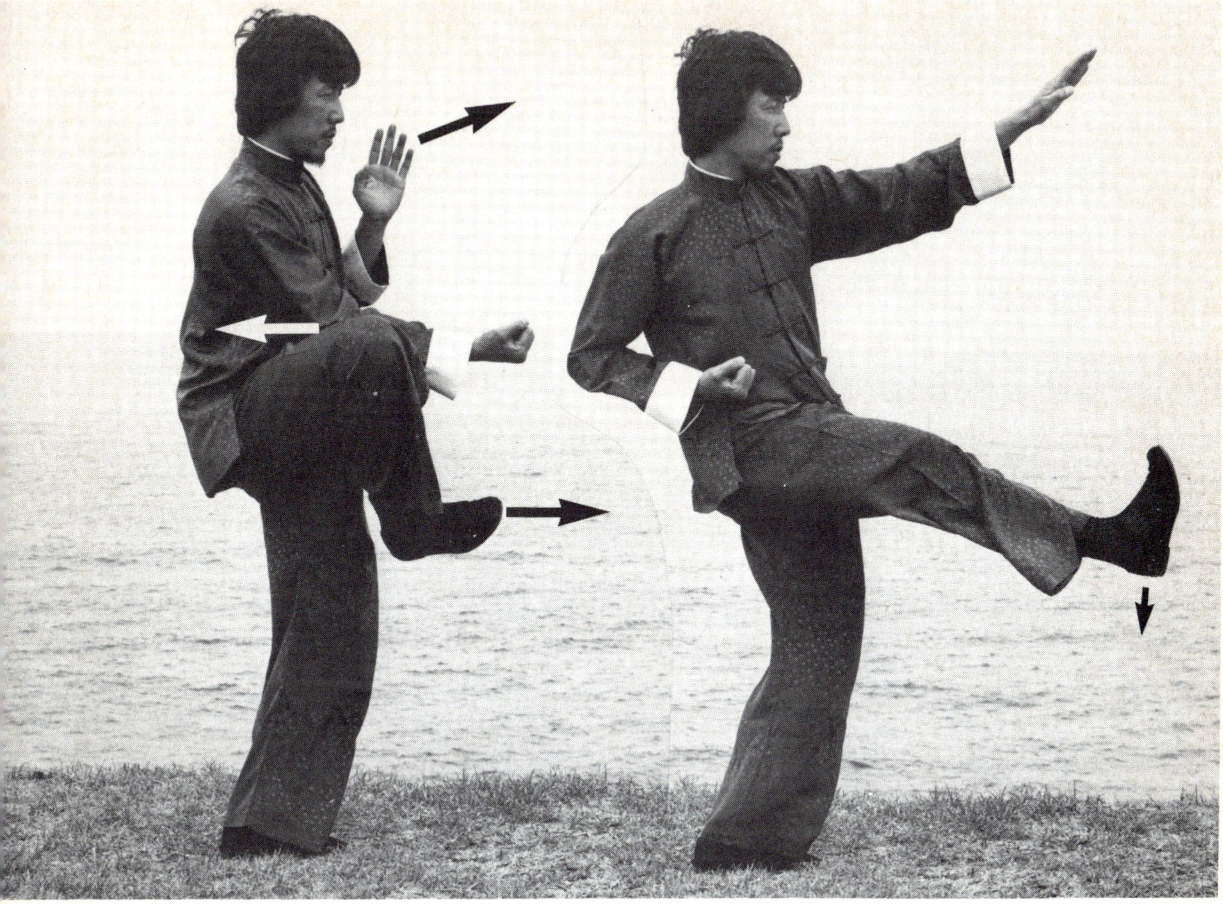

Arm movements

Turn your left palm to face the floor, then extend your left arm to jab with your fingers. Pull your right fist in to your right hip.

Co-ordination

From **Cross deflection** shift your body weight over to the left leg and turn your left palm to face the ground. Raise your right knee, and as you kick, jab with your left palm and pull in your right fist.

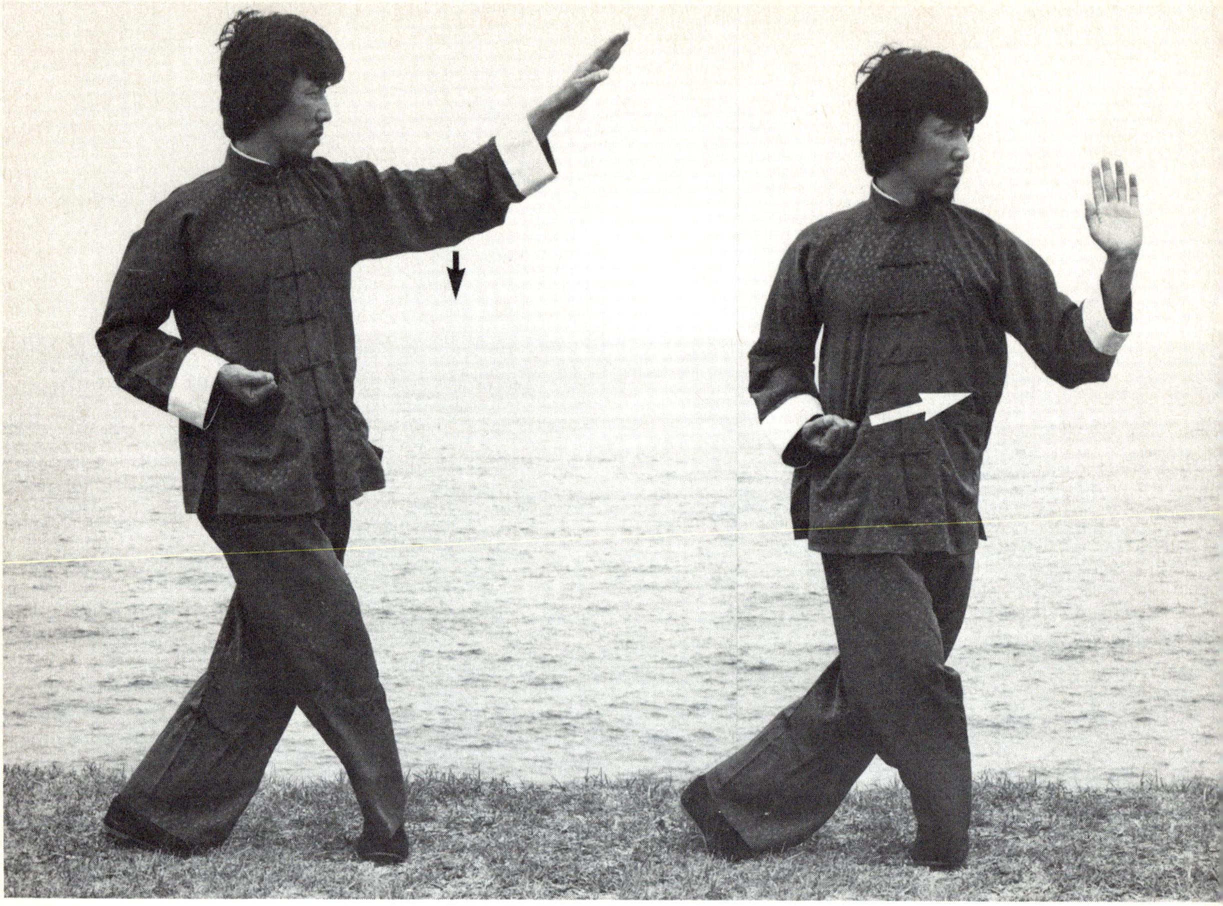

Step and parry

Footwork

Following through with the kicking momentum, allow the right foot to land in front.

Arm movements

Drop your left hand to parry as you twist your body to the right.

Co-ordination

From **Kick and thrust** follow through the kick, and step down with your right foot. Drop your left arm to parry as you twist your body to the right.

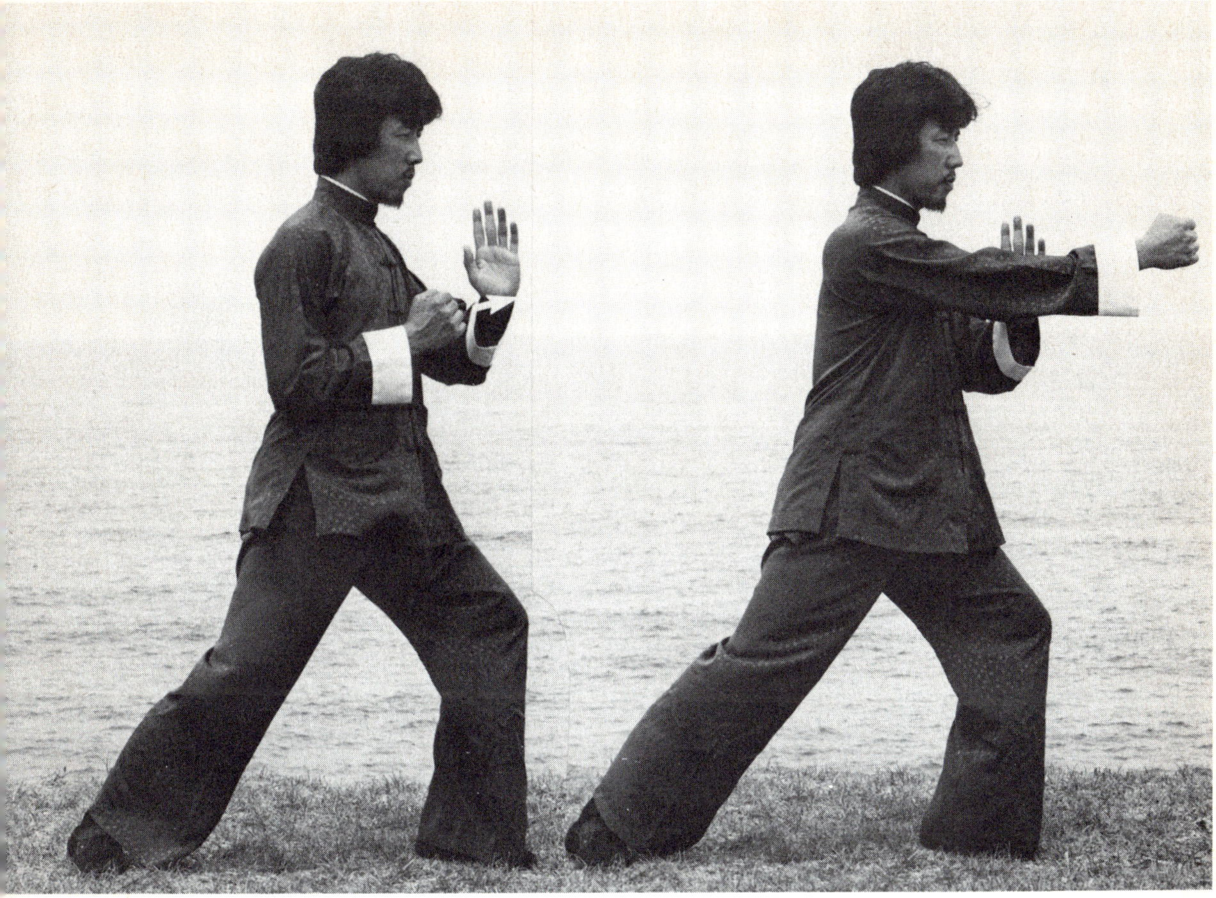

Punch

Footwork

Step forward to the left with your left foot. Turn your body to the left and shift your weight over to the left leg.

Arm movements

Deliver a punch with your right fist.

Co-ordination

From **Step and parry** step forward to the left with your left foot. Twist your body back to the left as you deliver a punch with your right fist, co-ordinating the punch with the body weight being shifted forward to the left leg.

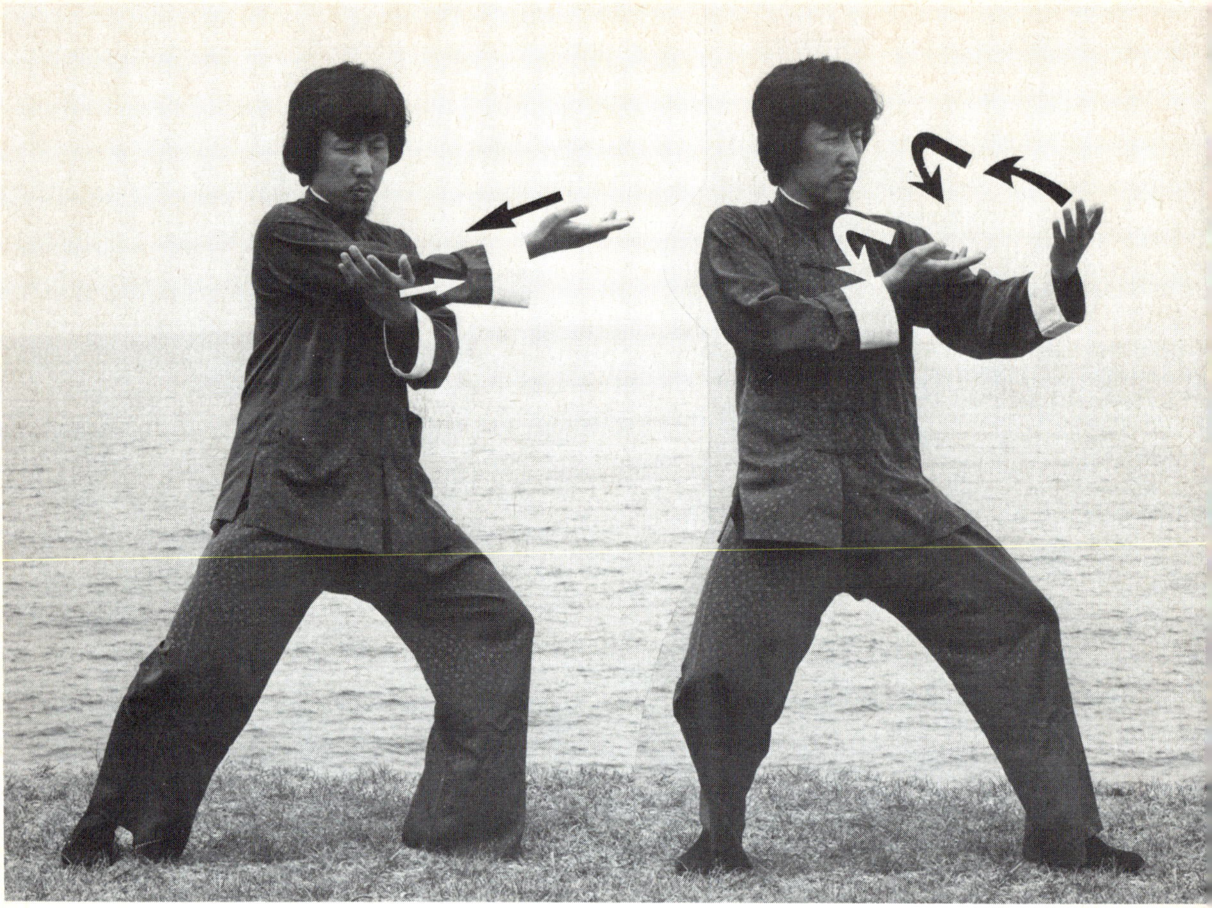

Closing the door

Footwork

Shift your weight back to the right leg, turning your shoulder to the right. Turn your shoulder back to the left and transfer the weight to your left foot.

Arm movements

Place your left palm under the right elbow, palm facing upwards. Draw your right arm back. Extend both arms to push.

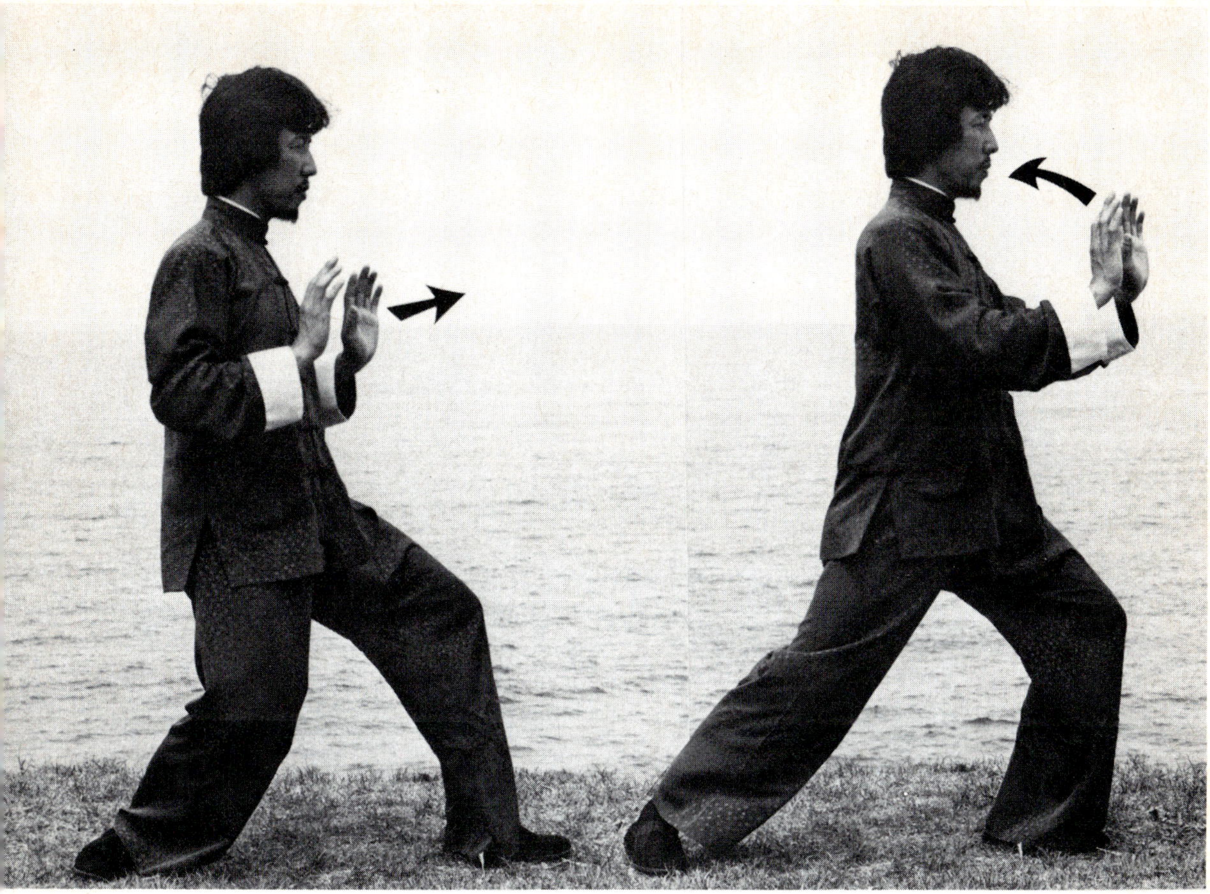

Co-ordination

From **Punch** place your left palm under the right elbow, and draw your right arm back as you turn your shoulder to the right and shift your body weight to the right leg. Then turning your shoulder back to the left, extend both arms to push, co-ordinating with the body weight being shifted forward to the left leg.

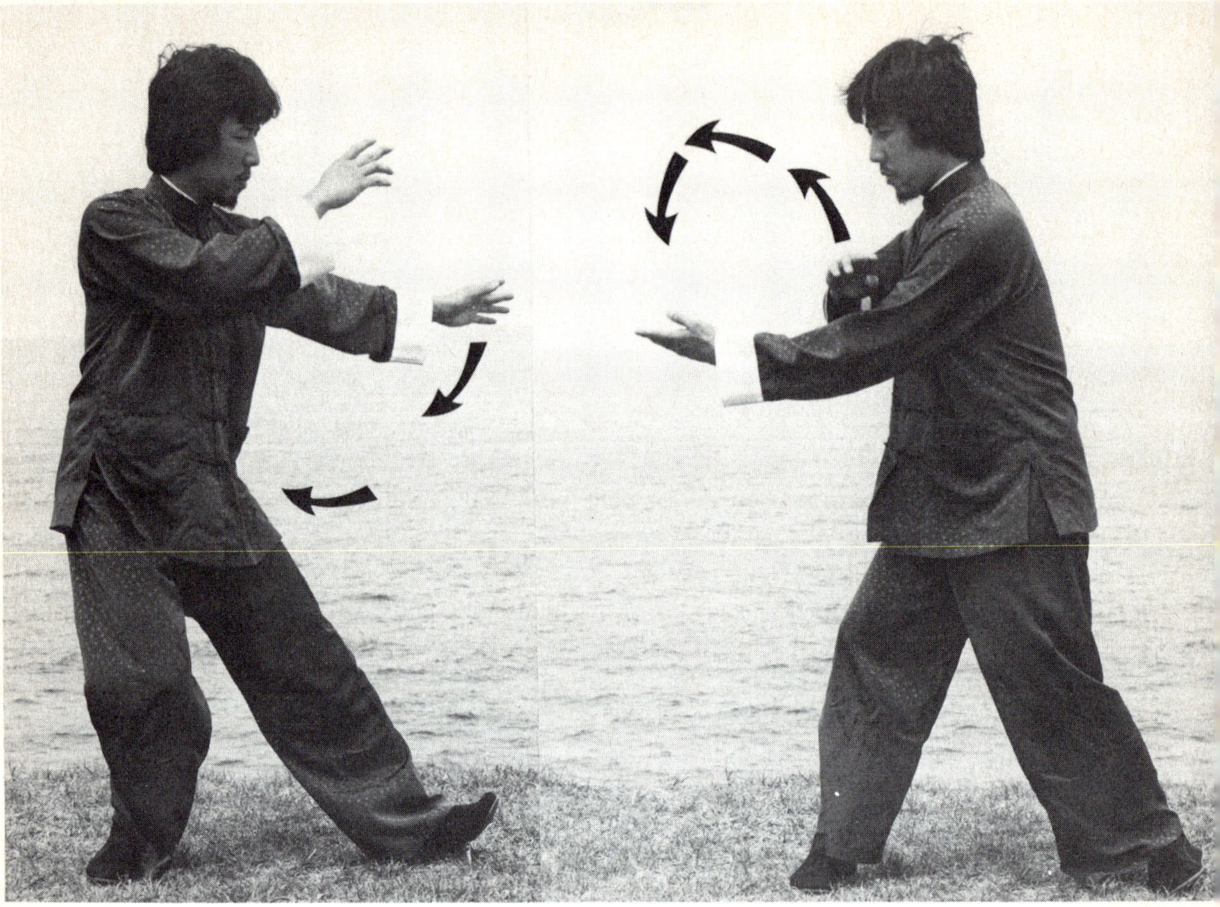

Cross hands

Footwork

Shift your weight back to your right leg. Raise your left toe, and pivoting on your left heel, turn your body 90 degrees to the right. Shift your body weight over to your left leg, and pivoting on your right toe, rotate your body 90 degrees to the left. Again rotate your body 90 degrees to the right, and step backwards with your right foot so that both feet are now parallel again.

Arm movements

Sweep your left arm down in an anti-clockwise arc to the back, and then up to the front, terminating at chest level. Sweep your right arm down to the back in a clockwise arc, and circling up to the front form a cross with the left hand.

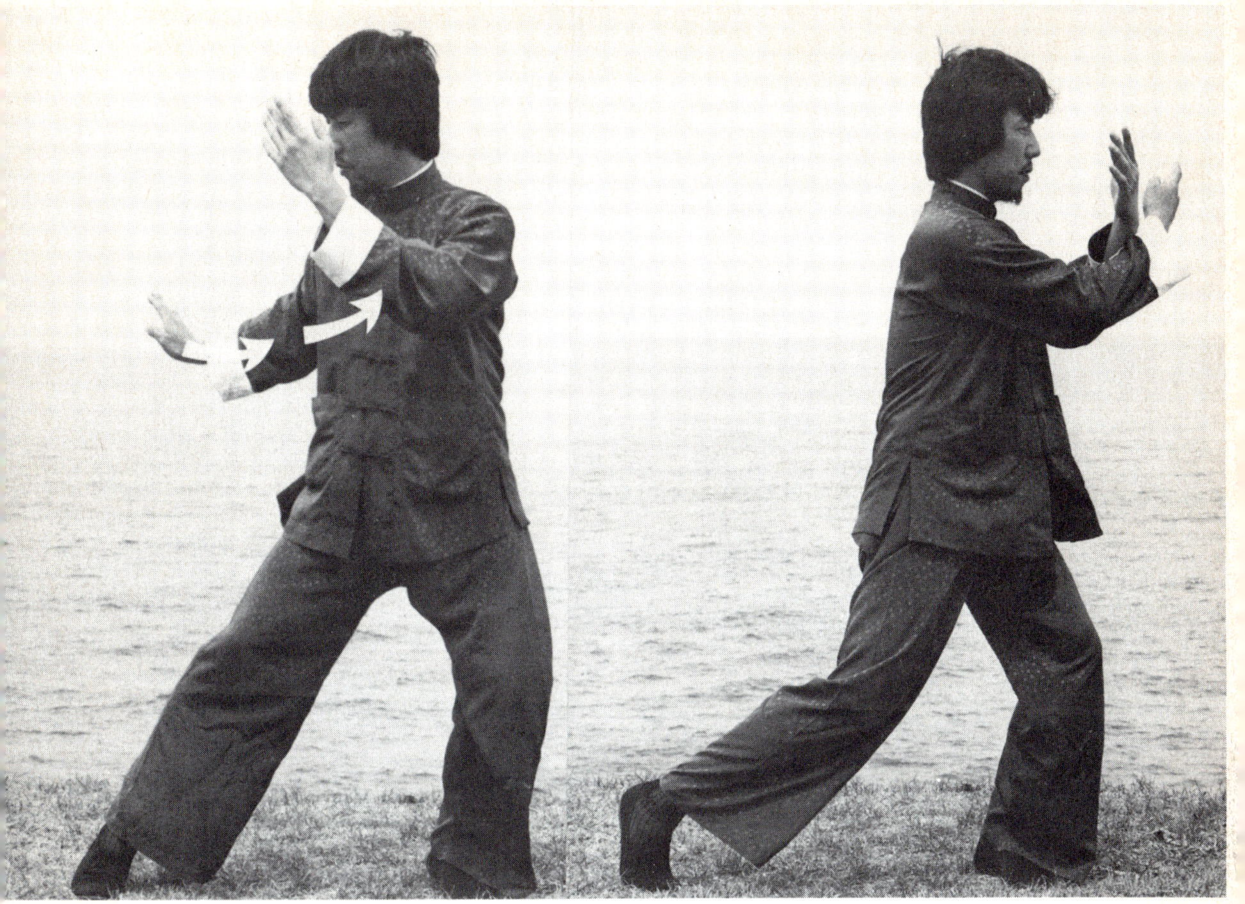

Co-ordination

From **Closing the door** shift your body weight back to your right leg, and pivot on your left heel. Sweep your left arm down to the back to scoop up to your chest, and turn your body 90 degrees to the right. Transfer your body weight over to your left leg, and pivot on your right toe. Now sweep your right arm down the right side of your body to scoop up to the front, forming a cross with your left hand. At the same time, turn your body 90 degrees to the left. Then turn your body 90 degrees back to the right, and step backwards with your right foot to bring your feet in line again.

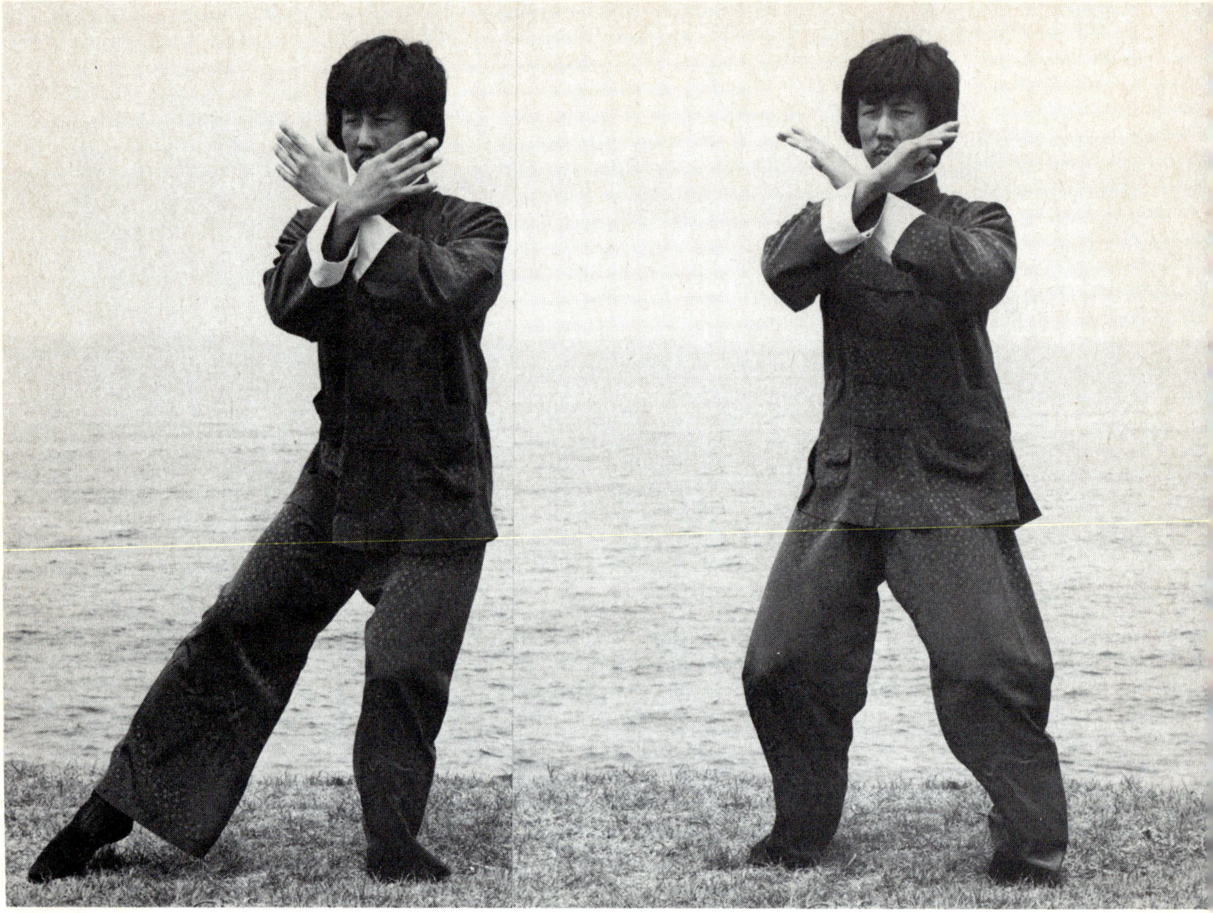

Closing the set

Separate both hands. Press your palms down to your sides as you rise to a normal standing position. Your posture is the same as the first posture, **Preparation.** You have now completed the first section of the Tai Chi set.

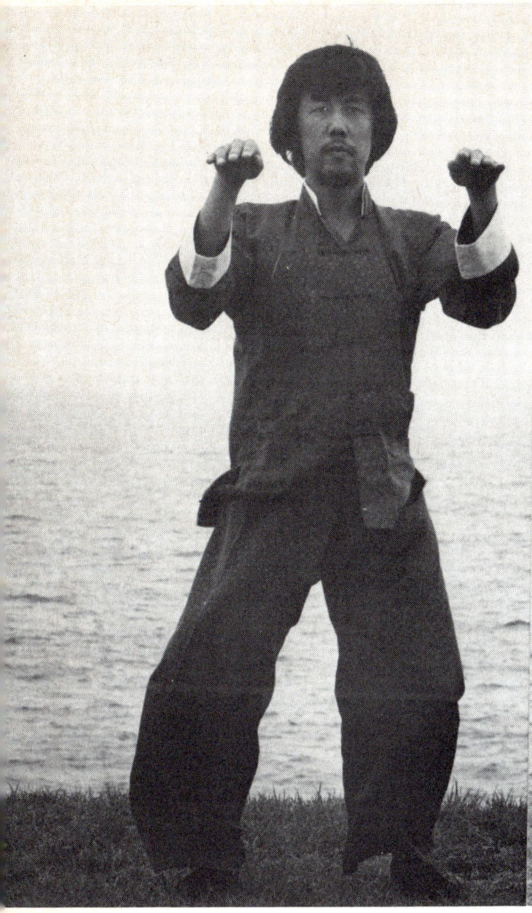
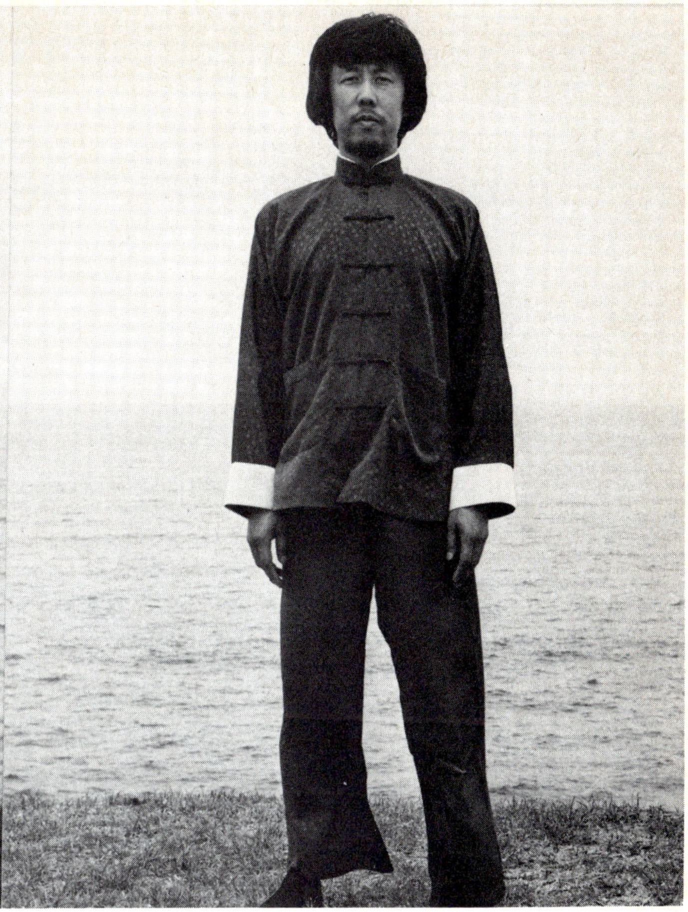

TAOIST ENERGY MEDITATION

The second exercise system is called Chinese Yoga or Taoist Energy Meditation.

Although this art can be practised on its own, traditionally it is used as a supplementary system to complement Tai Chi. Because of its semi-mobile nature, it is often referred to as ''semi-static meditation''.

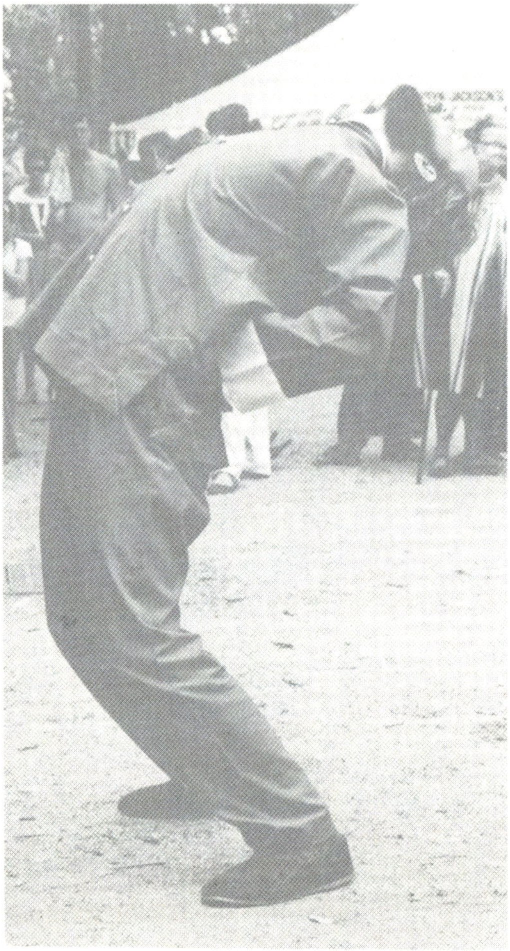

What is Taoist Energy Meditation

It is a meditation art based on gentle body stretching, diaphragmatic breathing and energy circulation. It consists of eight different exercises called The Eight Golden Treasures, each one designed to exercise and massage the internal organs. **Taoist Energy Meditation** is used as a preventive measure against sickness and disease, and to strengthen the body, mind and spirit.

Generally we tend to forget about our internal organs because they are hidden, and only become aware of them when they malfunction. The lungs are subjected to unending punishment from cigarette tar, petrol fumes, industrial pollution etc. Extreme pressures are put onto the heart through bad diet and stressful living. Research by the National Heart Foundation reveals that more than 30,000 people die of heart attack in this country each year. Similar examples can be found for the abuse and mutilation of the liver and kidneys.

The Taoists, realising the importance of proper maintenance of the internal organs, devised special yogic techniques to exercise and massage them.

Taoist Energy Meditation.

Table of exercises

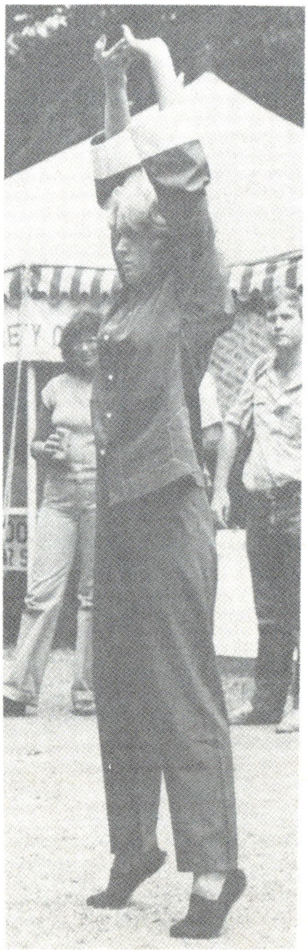

How to Practice the Eight Golden Treasures

In the performance of the exercises the following points should be observed:

1. The body should be loose and relaxed so that the Chi may circulate throughout the body.
2. The legs must be firmly rooted to the ground and the spine kept erect in the central position.
3. Breathing should be natural and co-ordinated with the stretching and bending movements.
4. Breathe only through your nostrils and direct the breath deep down into the tan tien. Place your tongue gently against the palate or roof of your mouth.

WARNING *Do not force or over-reach your own body's capability. Only proceed as far as it is comfortable for you.*

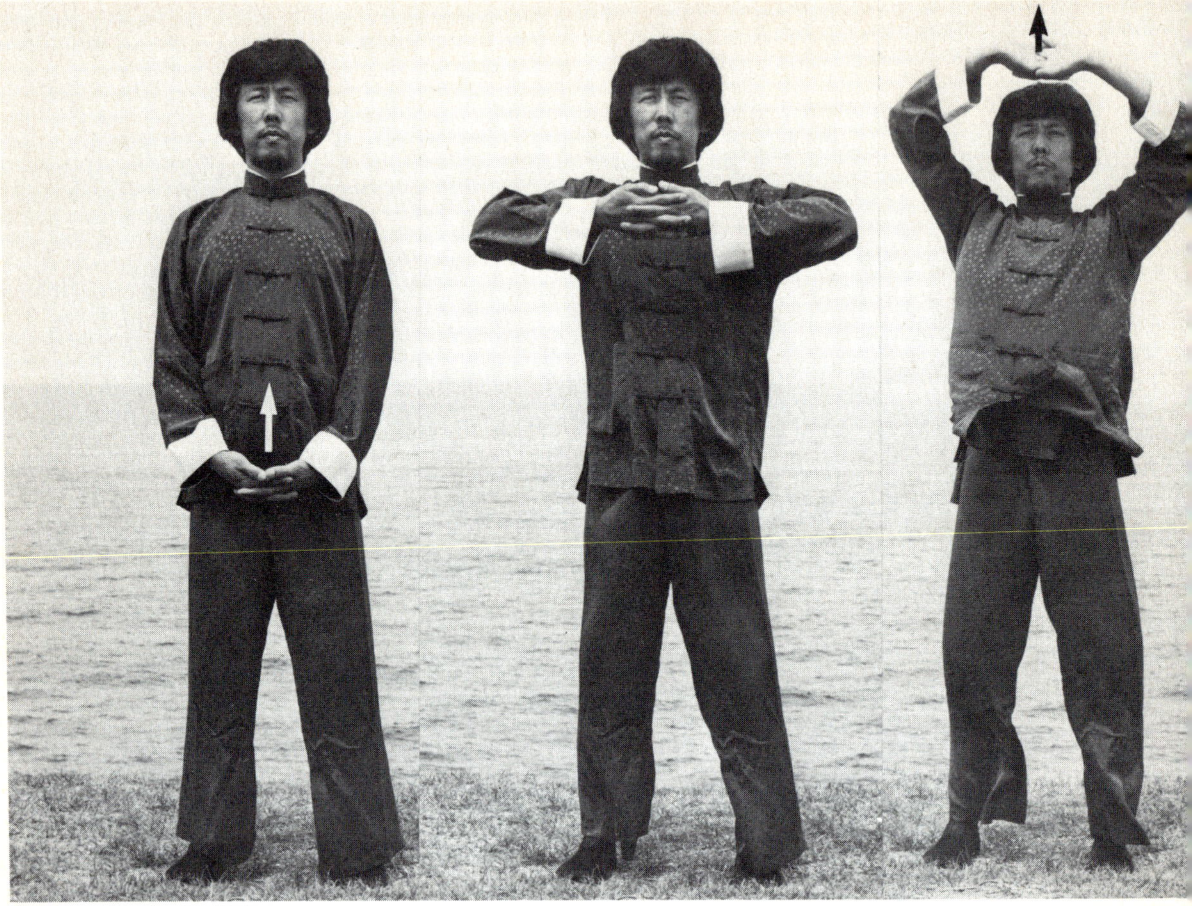

The Heavenly Lift

Imagery: Reach out with both hands to hold up the sky.

Exercise:

1. Stand comfortably at ease, with legs about shoulder width apart. Interlock your fingers and hold them in front of your abdomen, palms facing upwards.
2. Breathe in slowly as you raise your locked fingers up to your chest. Rotate your palms outwards as you push them out over your head in a stretching motion. As you do this, raise your heels and stand on your toes.
3. Exhale as you rotate your palms inward and lower them back to your abdomen. At the same time, lower your heels back down to the ground.
4. Repeat the exercise eight times.

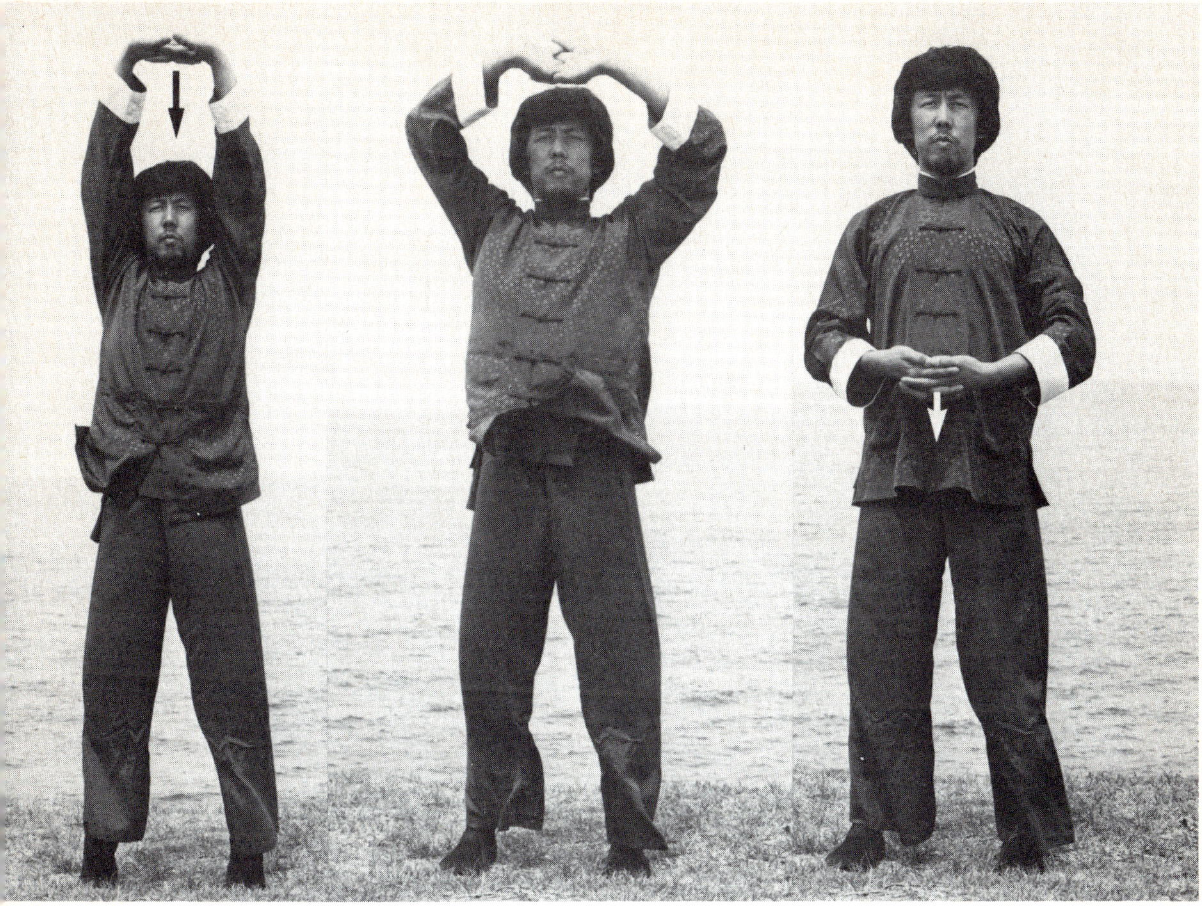

Function: Physically, this exercise improves the overall elasticity of the whole body. It lengthens ligaments, stretches the rib cage upwards, and strengthens the abdominal muscles. The movements provide excellent exercise for the various joints in the arms.

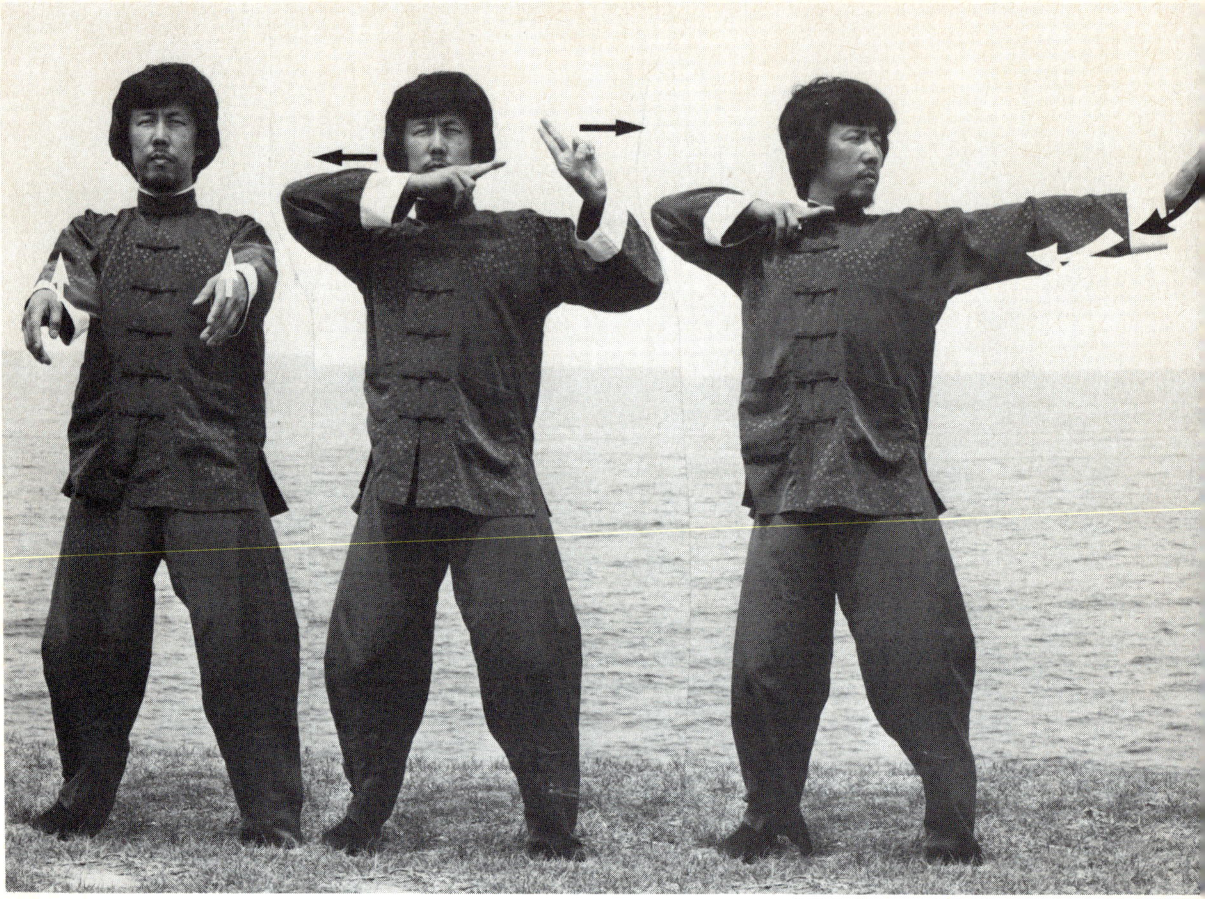

The Taoist Archer

Imagery: The archer lifts his bow, loads the arrow, draws the string to aim and lets fly the arrow to seek its target.

Exercise:

1. With legs about shoulder width apart bend your knees to lower yourself into a ‘‘riding horse’’ posture.
2. Breathe in slowly as you rotate to aim to the left; extending to stretch your left (bow) arm, and retracting to draw the string with your right (arrow) arm.
3. Exhale slowly as you release the arrow. Rotating back to the front, lower your arms to the side of your body.
4. Repeat the exercise for the right side of the body, reversing the bow and arrow hands.
5. Repeat eight times, four for each side.

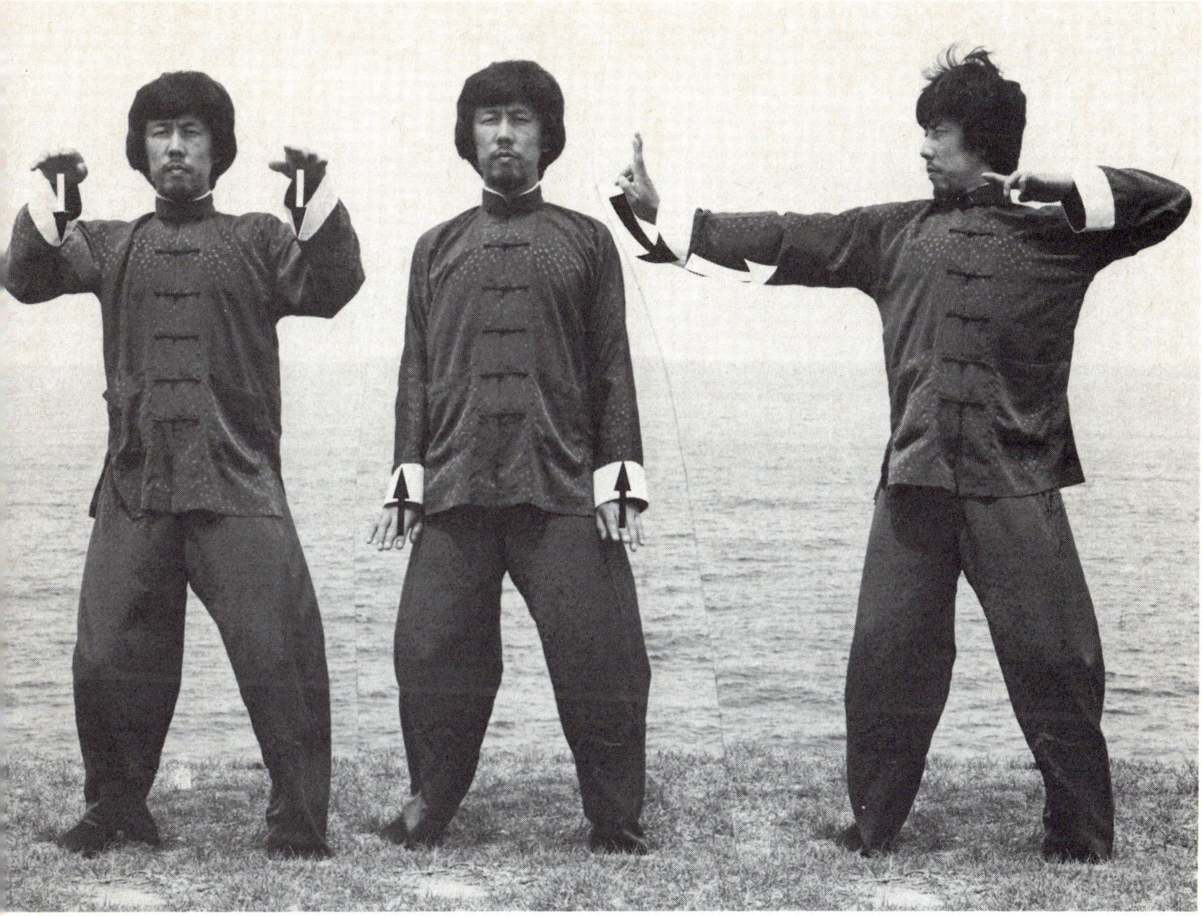

Function: Externally, to improve the elasticity and muscle tone of the arms and shoulders. Internally to enhance the respiratory system.

In this exercise, the movements stretch the rig cage sideways, which expands the chest and increases the lung capacity. This is further assisted by the downward motion of the diaphragm through the Chi being mentally directed to the tan tien.

The resulting internal pressures created by these movements massage the heart, liver, lungs and intestines. In particular the blood circulation and oxygen intake are vastly increased. This improved respiration refreshes the whole body and renews the energy supply.

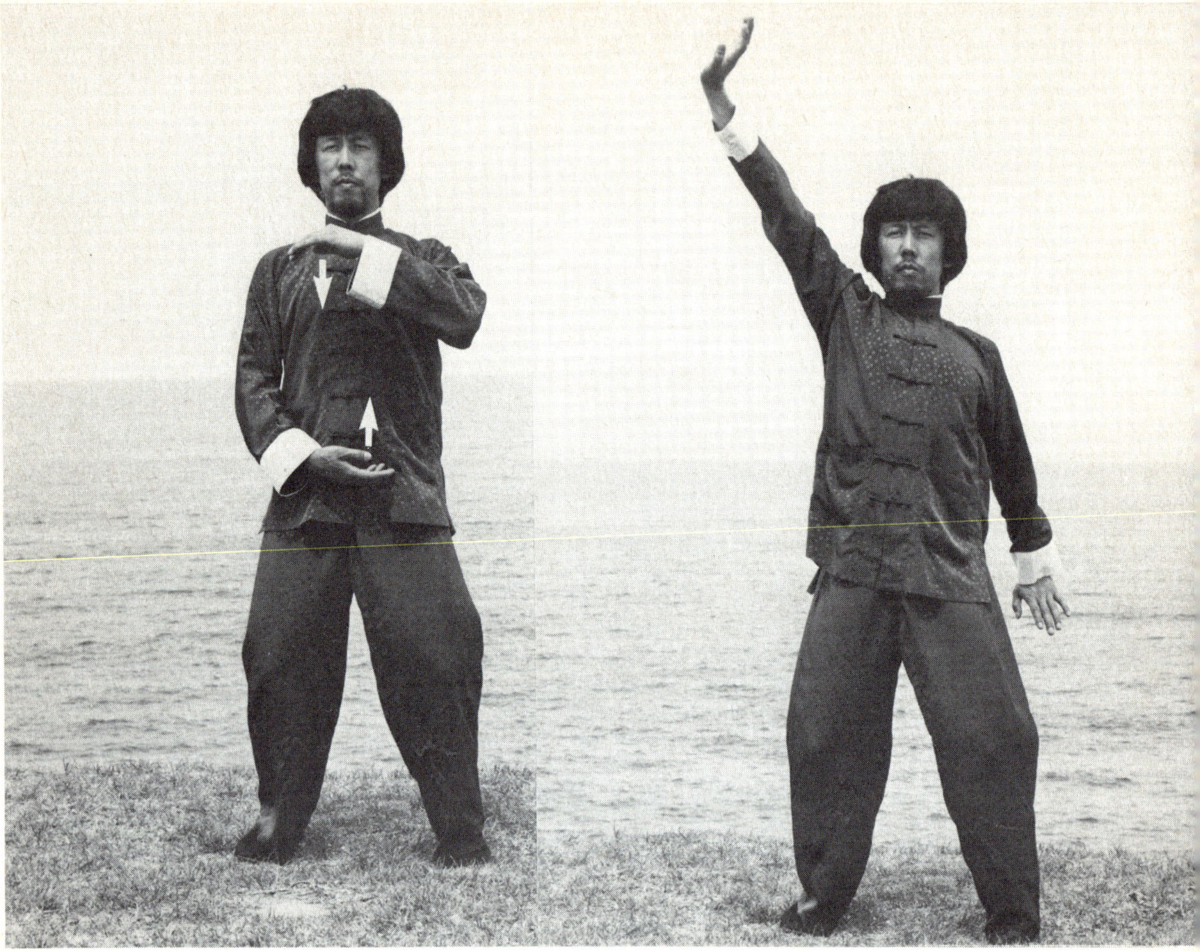

White Crane Spreads Wings

Imagery: In the morning sun stands the majestic crane. Unfolding, it spreads its wings; one upwards to the sky, the other downwards to the earth.

Exercise:

1. Stand with legs apart in the ''riding horse'' posture. Raise your arms to hold an imaginary ball in front of your abdomen; left palm facing downwards on top of the ball, right palm facing upwards supporting the ball.

2. Inhale slowly as you spread your arms in opposite directions; right palm pushing outwards to the sky, left palm pressing downwards to the earth.

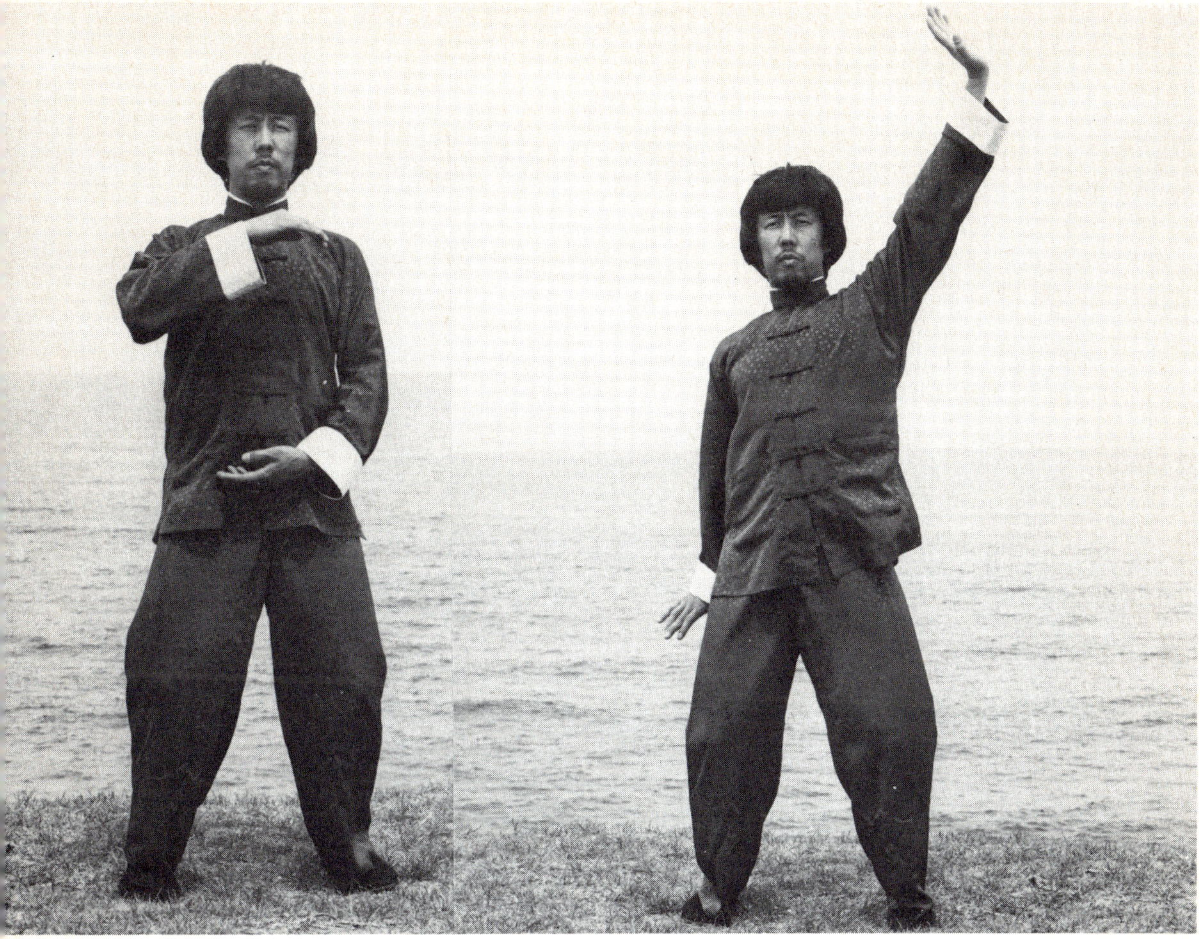

3. Exhale slowly as you return your arms to the holding ball posture. The positions of the palms are now reversed; left palm supporting the ball and right palm on top of the ball.
4. Repeat the exercise for the other side of the body.
5. Repeat eight times, four times for each side alternately.

Function: The two way stretch strengthens the ligaments of the arms and shoulder. The stretching movements exercise the spleen and stomach, thereby enhancing the digestive system.

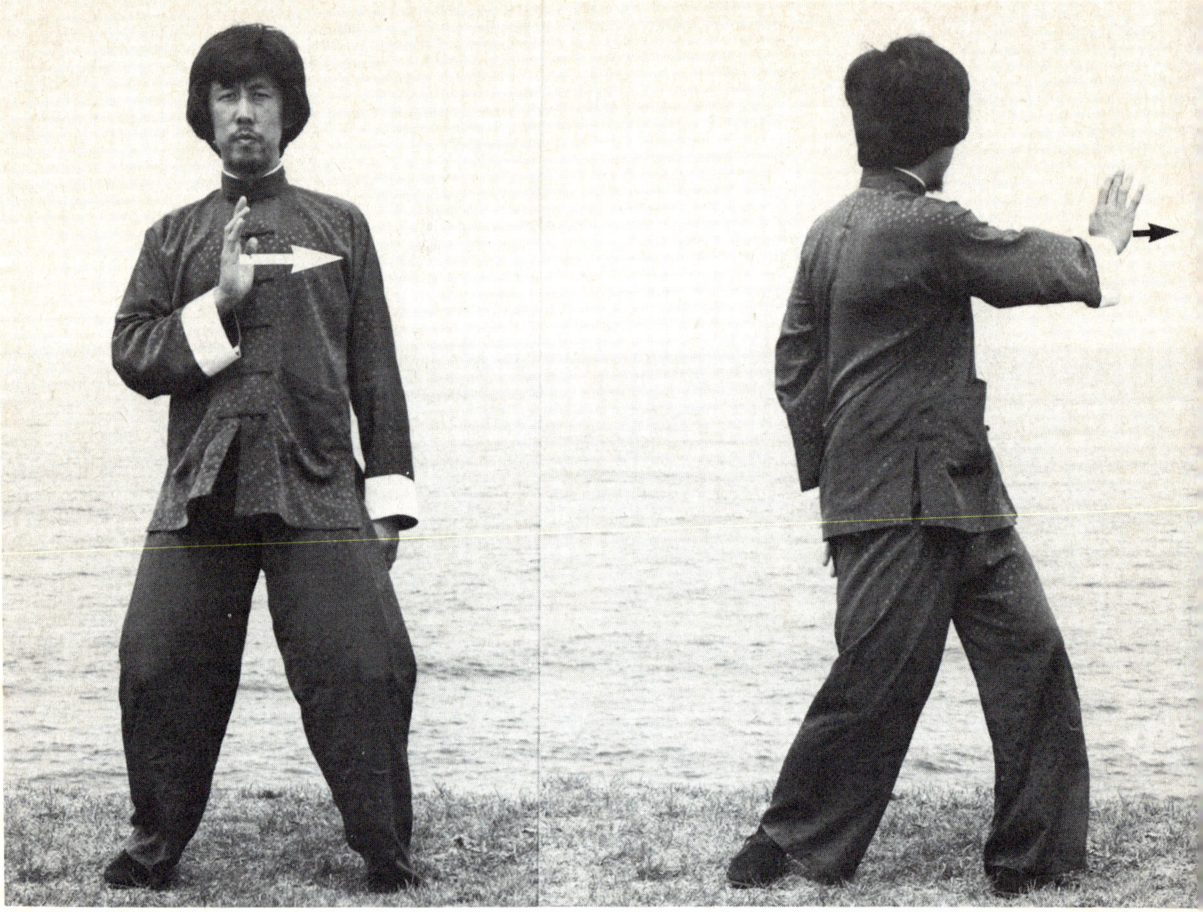

The Spinal Twist

Imagery: Picture your spinal column as the central axis on which your body turns.

Exercise:

1. Sit in "riding horse" posture. Inhale as you bring your right hand into a prayer posture in front of your chest.
2. Exhale slowly as you rotate 180 degrees to the left. Extend your right palm to press out as far as possible.
3. Inhale as you rotate back to the original position. At the same time retract your right arm to the side of your body and bring your left hand into the prayer posture in front of your chest.
4. Repeat the movement on the other side.
5. Repeat the movements eight times, four for each side alternately.

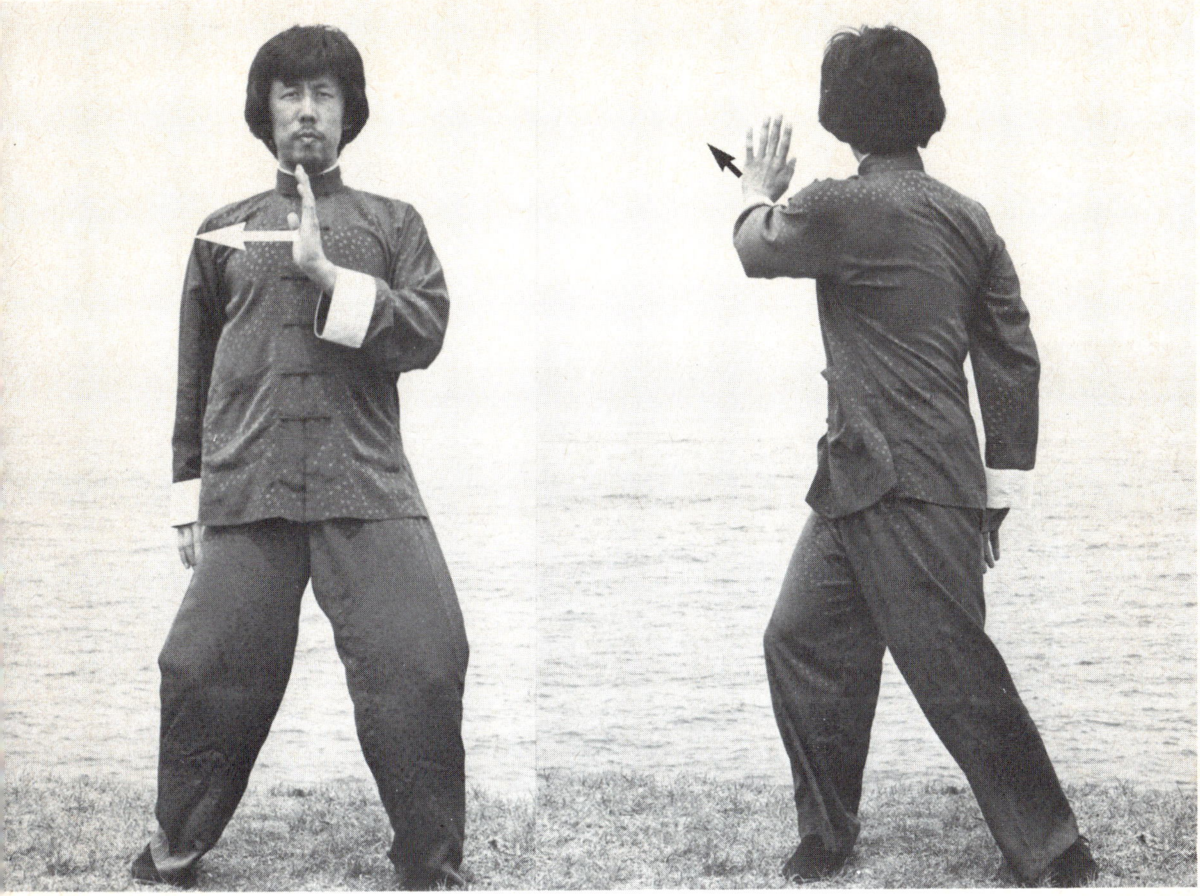

Function: This exercise stretches the front and back muscles, and produces a massaging effect on the nervous system, thereby stimulating overall energy flow. It further develops and strengthens the lungs, improving the respiratory system.

Physically, it improves the tone of the neck, chest, shoulder and abdominal muscles, and reduces the waist line.

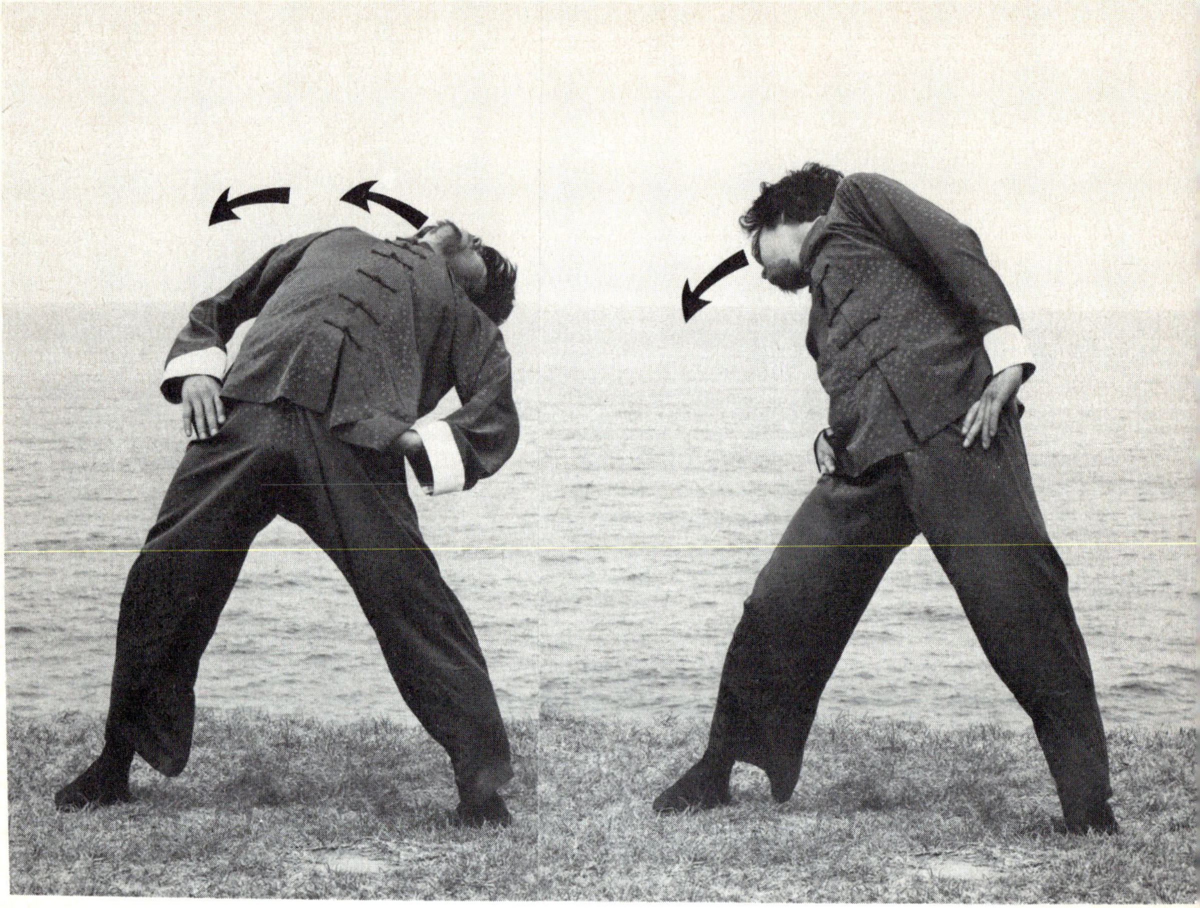

The Rotary Waist

Imagery: Shake your head, wriggle your tail and release the heart's fire.

Exercise:

1. Sit in "riding horse" stance, hands gripping the thighs.
2. Inhale as you bring your head up to circle anti-clockwise to the back.
3. Exhale as you bend down to your right to circle past your front to the left.

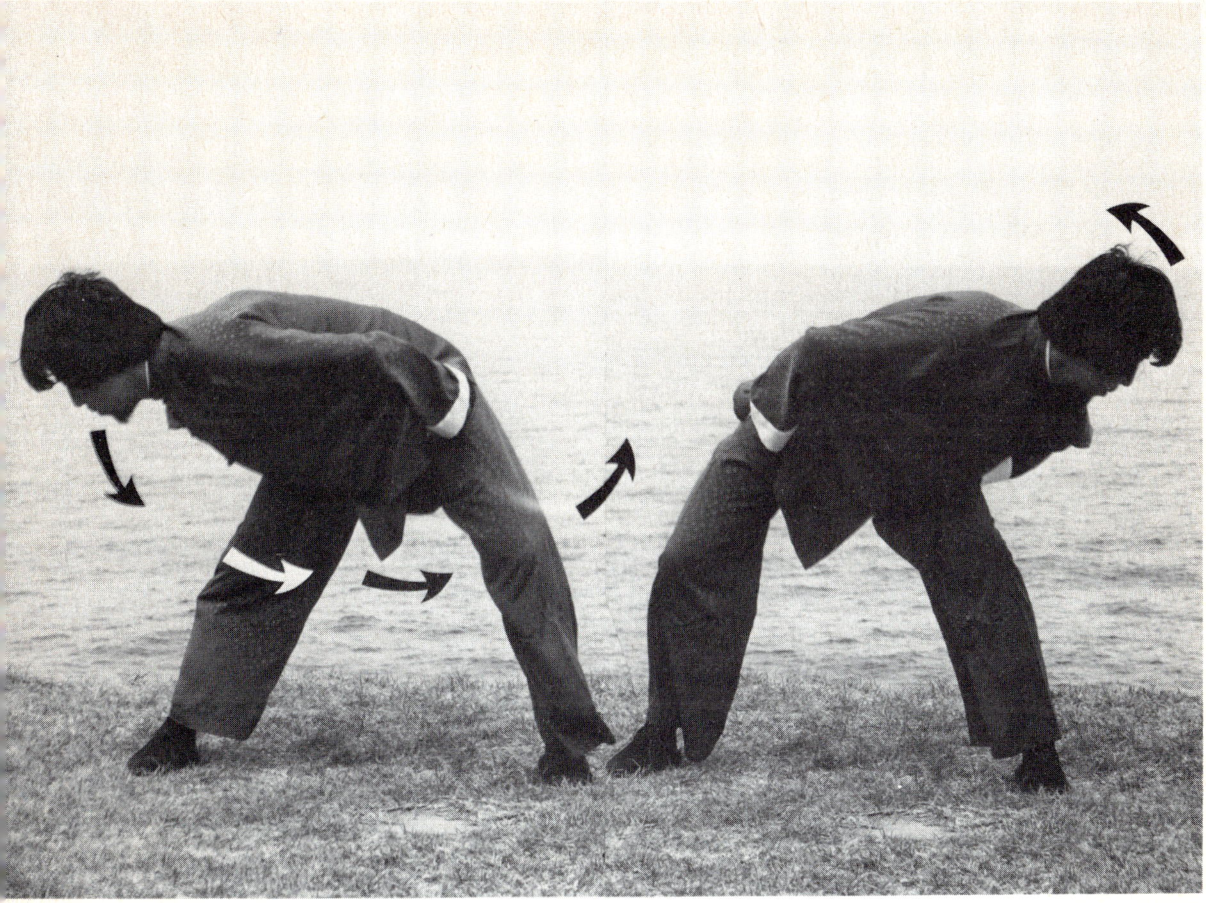

4. Reverse the direction and repeat the whole exercise eight times; four for each side alternately.

Function: Physically it reduces the waistline and strengthens the abdominal muscles. Physiologically, it improves the digestive and circulatory systems. It stimulates the overall energy flow and relieves emotional energy blockage.

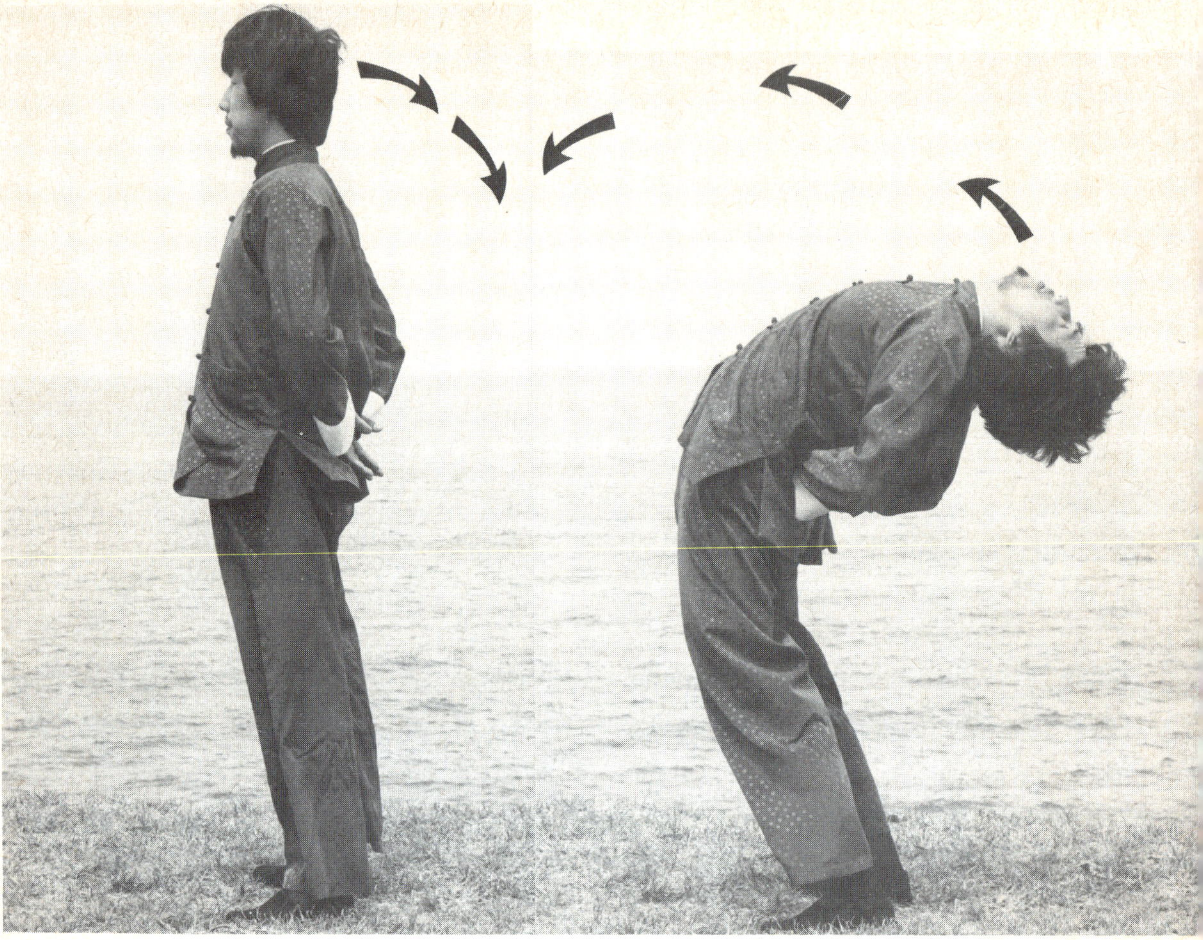

Kidney and Spinal Bend

Exercise:

1. Stand erect with feet shoulder width apart. Rest the back of your wrists against your kidneys.
2. Inhale slowly and bend backwards as far as possible.
3. Exhale slowly as you straighten and bend forward to grip your toes.

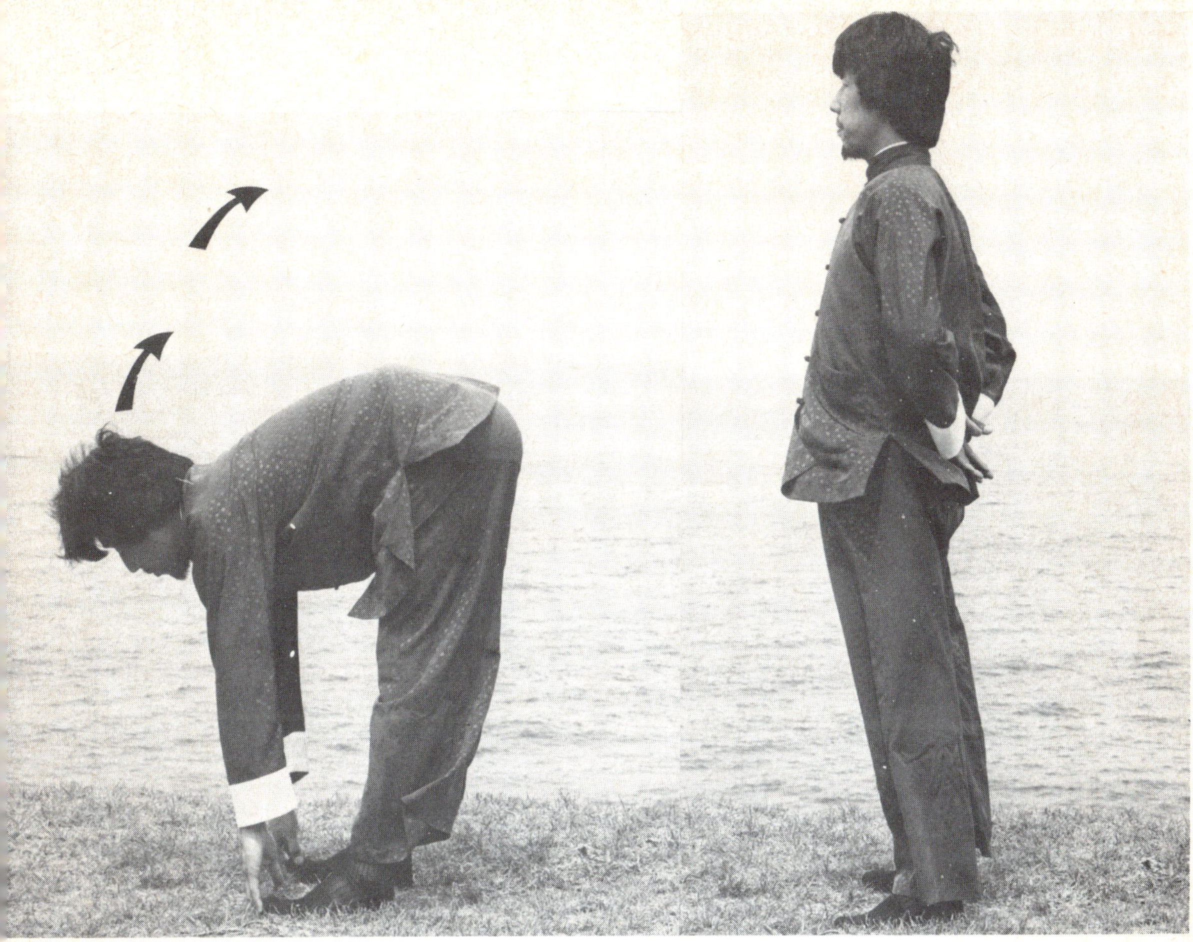

4. Repeat eight times.

Function: This exercise increases the elasticity and tone of the abdominal muscles and flexibility of the spine. Physiologically, it stimulates the kidneys and improves toxic waste expulsion.

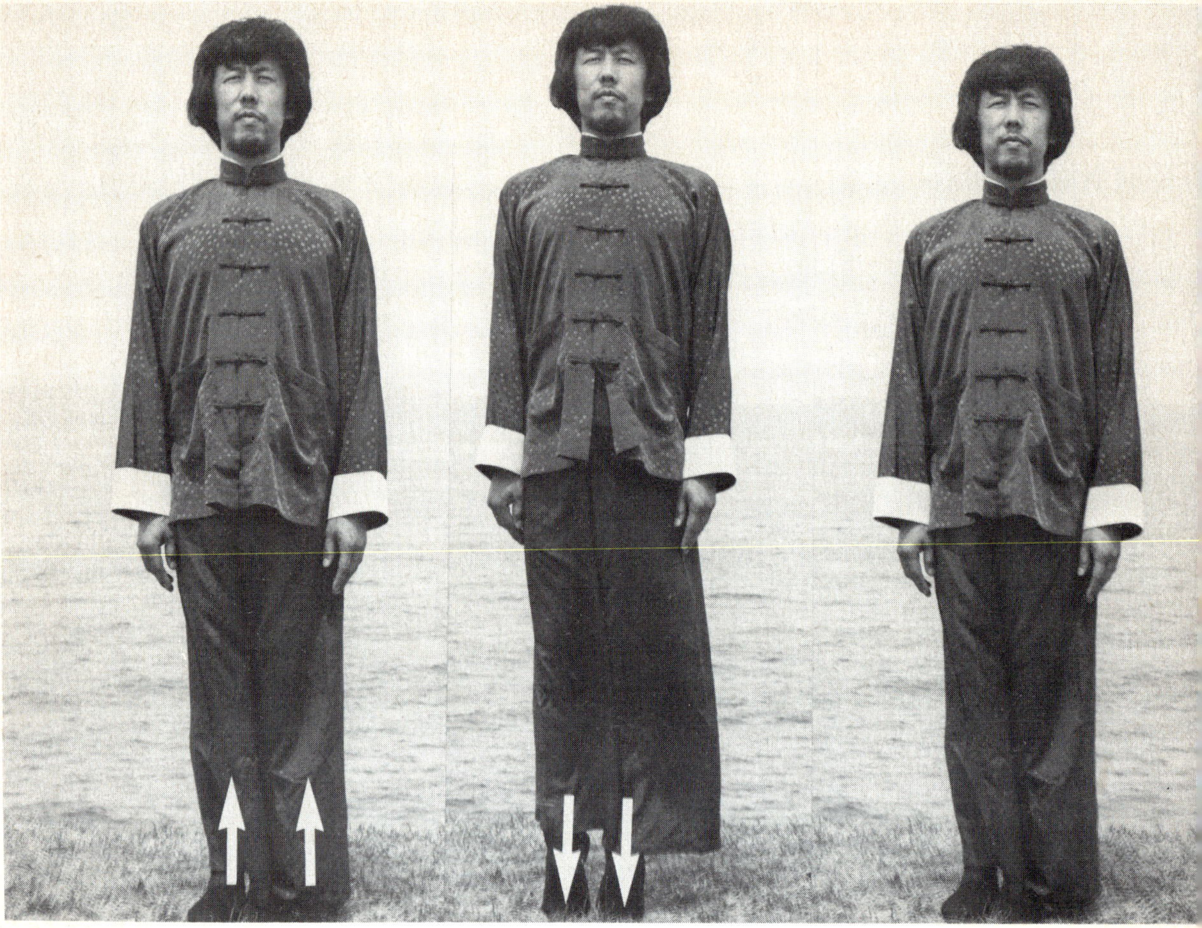

The Spinal Jolt

Exercise:

1. Stand erect with feet together, arms hanging by your sides.
2. Inhale slowly as you raise your heels to stand on your toes.
3. Exhale as you drop your heels back to the ground in a gentle slamming jolt.
3. Repeat eight times.

Function: The jolting vibration stimulates the central nervous system which benefits all the internal organs. Physically it strengthens the leg muscles.

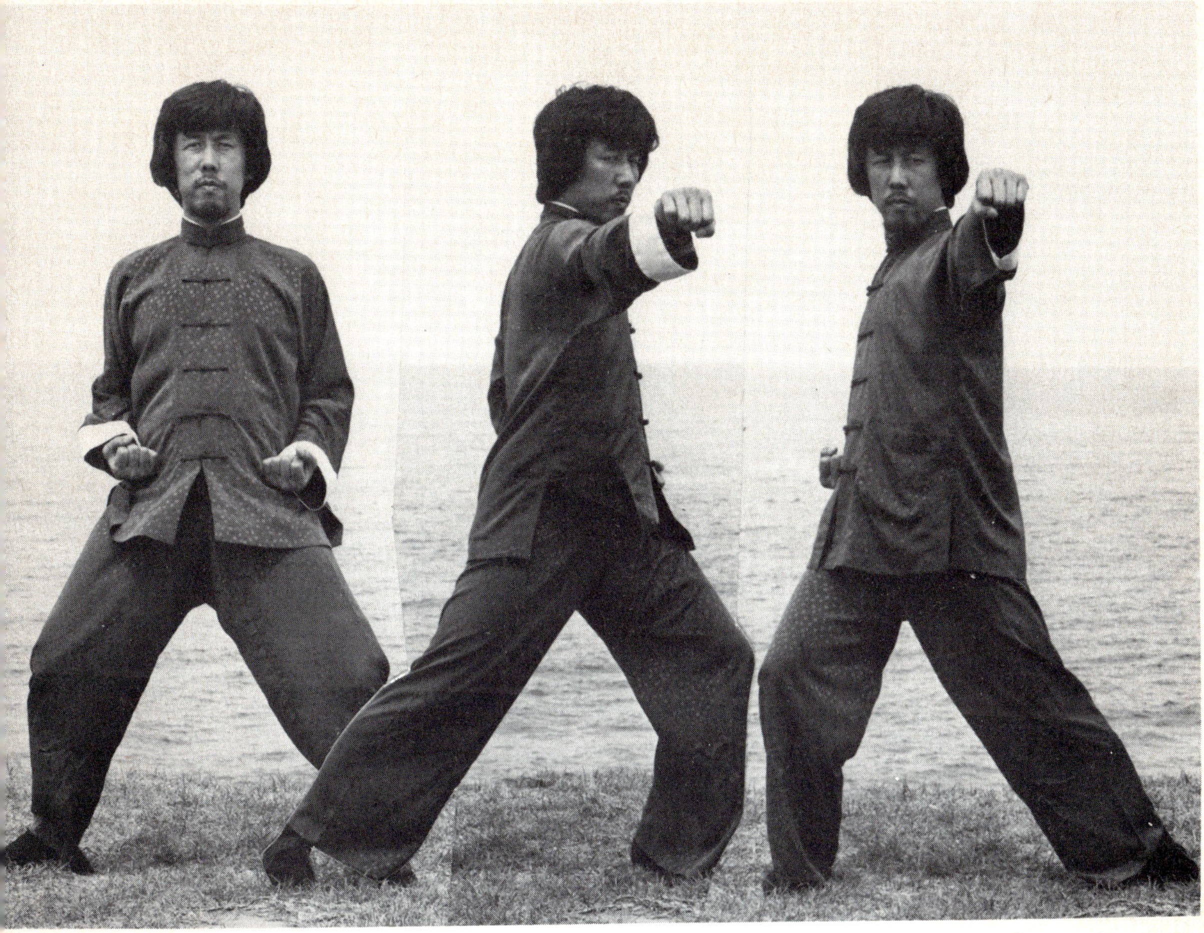

The Angry Fists

Imagery: Shadow boxing by throwing imaginary punches.

Exercise:

1. With legs apart, lower into ''riding horse'' posture. Open eyes wide to gaze ahead.
2. Inhale slowly and draw both fists to your waist.
3. Exhale as you rotate to the left. At the same time extend your right fist in an outward screwing motion.
4. Repeat movement for other side.
5. Repeat movement eight times, four for each side alternately.

Function: Improves and strengthens eyesight, arms, shoulders and legs. This exercise stimulates energy flow which enhances blood circulation and refreshes body cells.

CONCLUSION

The end of this book is the beginning of the next phase for you. I have presented only the very basics of Tai Chi in its simplest form for the beginner. If it has interested you enough to spur you to further exploration, then a whole new world of intriguing Chinese culture awaits you.

The Chinese have protected their knowledge well, but now that it is available a new phase of the art must surely begin. Although Tai Chi originated in China it is such a versatile art that it must surely be adopted internationally and benefit everyone. Whether it is practised as a dance form, a martial art or just plain physical exercise, its natural philosophy will guide its exponents to a healthier life style and a deeper appreciation of our eco-system.

The most successful method is to use it as a daily ritual, entrenching it as a habit from the early period of dedicated enthusiasm.

As a body-mind integration system, the art possesses all the ingredients to absorb one's total concentration. It only requires that little bit of dedication through regular practice for you to experience its special feeling of enlightenment — this is the reward of the dedicated student.

The aesthetic quality of Tai Chi lies not in its visual experience but in the feel of it, on the inside, for the person who does it. It is like the pearl within the jewel case.

It is said that the highest ideal of Chinese culture is a person with a sense of detachment towards life — a person with a sense of wise disenchantment. Whatever your reason for learning Tai Chi, adopt a sense of fun and play, and above all enjoy the experience. We have a saying in Chinese — "play me a set of Tai Chi".